Homeopathy for midwives

Editorial advisors: Denise Tiran, UK, Ellen Philpot, USA, and Deanne Williams, USA

For Churchill Livingstone

Commissioning editor: Inta Ozols
Project manager: Valerie Burgess
Project development editor: Dinah Thom
Design direction: Judith Wright
Project controller: Pat Miller
Illustrator: Robert Britton
Copy editor: Holly Regan-Jones
Indexer: Tarrant Ranger Indexing Agency
Sales promotion executive: Hilary Brown

Homeopathy for midwives

Barbara Geraghty BA LicLCCH RSHom
Registered Homeopath, London, UK

Introduction by
Denise Tiran RGN RM ADM PGCEA
Principal Lecturer in Complementary Therapies and Midwifery,
University of Greenwich, London, UK

Foreword by
Lesley Page MSc BA RM RN RMT RNT
The Queen Charlotte's Professor of Midwifery Practice,
The Centre for Midwifery Practice and Policy,
The Wolfson School of Health Science,
Thames Valley University, London, UK

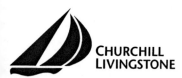
**CHURCHILL
LIVINGSTONE**

NEW YORK EDINBURGH LONDON MADRID MELBOURNE SAN FRANCISCO AND TOKYO 1997

Churchill Livingstone
An imprint of Elsevier Science Limited

First published 1997
Transferred to digital printing 2002

ISBN 0 443 05708 7

British Library Cataloguing in Publication Data
A catalogue record for this book is available from the British Library.

Library of Congress Cataloging in Publication Data
A catalog record for this book is available from the Library of Congress.

Note
Medical knowledge is constantly changing. As new information
becomes available, changes in treatment, procedures, equipment and
the use of drugs become necessary. The authors and publishers have, as
far as it is possible, taken care to ensure that the information given in
this text is accurate and up to date. However, readers are strongly
advised to confirm that the information, especially with regard to drug
usage, complies with latest legislation and standards of practice.

Contents

Foreword

About a decade ago I noticed with interest that local Royal College of Midwives meetings that featured homeopathy drew crowds of midwives, whereas other meetings survived on the faithful few. Even then, it seemed to me, there was a fundamental resonance between the principles and approaches of homeopathy and midwifery. At that time, the Winterton report (House of Commons 1992), and *Changing Childbirth* (Expert Maternity Group 1993), had not yet been published. However, even the seeds of the transformation that was to happen in the maternity services were sown. For example, new organizations of care were being developed, and midwives were starting to recognize limits to the 'treatments' they used. Many of these new organizations sought to allow midwives to care for the whole woman and the whole family. They encouraged midwives to evaluate their care, and to supplement the limited system of curative, allopathic and surgical treatments with more 'natural' forms of healing and help.

Having read *Homeopathy for Midwives*, it is clear why those sessions drew so much interest. It is clear from this book that the principles of homeopathy are indeed resonant with the principles of midwifery. Barbara Geraghty describes homeopathy as 'a system of healing which helps the natural tendency of the body to heal itself'. It is 'a person centred holistic approach, where people are seen not only in terms of their bodies but also in terms of their mind and spirit'. These are also the principles of midwifery.

Now, following the two government reports (the Winterton report and *Changing Childbirth*) on the maternity service, there are few who could have avoided rethinking their approach to care. These two reports have led to the creation of woman and family focused services. Professionals have been encouraged to recognize the profound effect of care around pregnancy, birth and the early weeks of life on human health and happiness.

In this way, professionals have been encouraged to rethink much of the routine care that has formed a large part of recent maternity services. This rethinking is moving us from many of the treatments of women and babies in current use: treatments that are based on an idea of the body as a mechanical assembly of separate systems. In short, midwives have now been given licence to establish a holistic woman-centred approach where women and their families are seen, as in homeopathy, 'not only in terms of their bodies, but also their minds and spirits'.

There are other parts of this book that run in parallel with good midwifery. *Homeopathy for Midwives* provides research evidence where it exists, but is honest about limitations and areas of uncertainty. At each step the midwife is cautioned not to go outside of the realms of her knowledge and expertise.

Homeopathy often seems mysterious, but this is partly because understanding requires a different mind set, and partly because homeopathy is complex. This book demystifies the subject and provides greater understanding. The book aims to help midwives become 'suitably conversant, confident and competent with homeopathy and able to advise a client who wants to make use of homeopathic remedies while in their care'.

This book will be invaluable for midwives. It provides detailed tables to guide the use of remedies, as well as a clear explanation of the history of homeopathy, the principles which underlie it, and the way homeopathy should be used. *Homeopathy for Midwives* will also provoke thought and ideas in the many midwives who already have an interest in the subject. Moreover, it may fill a gap for other midwives, who are generally aware of the limitations of the approaches of care and cure which dominate the present maternity services, and who are seeking to find complementary methods of treatment: treatments for the whole woman, baby and family. In short, there should be something in this book for all midwives.

1997   L.P.

REFERENCES

Expert Maternity Group 1993 Changing Childbirth: report of the
  Expert Maternity Group, Vol 1. HMSO, London
House of Commons 1992 Health Services Select Committee report on
  the maternity services. House of Commons, London

Preface

Homeopathy is a system of healing which helps to stimulate the natural tendency of the body to heal itself. It is a person-centred, 'holistic' approach, where people are seen not only in terms of their bodies but also in terms of their mind and spirit. Health is seen as the well-being of all three parts and ill health as dis-harmony within the whole person. Symptoms are the means of expressing this dis-harmony. The homeopathic prescriber examines each individual and her specific symptoms, with the result that two individuals may receive different remedies for the same medical diagnosis.

Homeopathy can be used safely in many situations before, during and after pregnancy to raise the general level of health and well-being of both mother and child. It can enhance normal labour, helping to minimize pain, discomfort and distress.

This work aims to help midwives to become suitably conversant, confident and competent with homeopathy and to be able to advise a client who wants to make use of homeopathic remedies while under their care.

1997   B.G.

Acknowledgements

I wish to thank Francis Treuherz, Rosemary Heed, John Churchill, Bridget Cummings and the late Ann Larkin for their enthusiasm and encouragement in the early days of this project.

Special thanks to Denise Tiran for her contribution and advice. I also wish to thank the various critics and correspondents who made constructive suggestions for alterations and improvements to the text. Thanks also to the team at Churchill Livingstone for their patience and support in my struggles as a first-time author. Many thanks to Stewart McOwen for his helpful reference suggestions.

Above all, thanks to my family, Barbara McCarthy and other close friends, without whose loyalty and understanding this work would not have been possible.

Part 1

Understanding and using homeopathy

Introduction

D. Tiran

Complementary and alternative therapies were, until recently, considered little short of witchcraft or quackery. However, their re-emergence in the health care arena around the world has been swift and dynamic until, today, they are increasingly being considered beneficial for a variety of conditions.

The expectations of the general public have grown and nowhere is this more apparent than in health care. Since the end of the Second World War, the health of nations in the Westernized world has improved dramatically. The advent of a vast array of new pharmaceutical preparations has reduced the incidence and severity of many life-threatening conditions and worldwide immunization programmes have virtually eradicated some diseases. In Europe, rebuilding and restoration following the destruction of the war years have resulted in improved standards of housing and sanitation while economic prosperity in both Europe and the USA has enabled the majority of people to enjoy a better standard of living. Developments in agricultural technology and refrigerated transportation mean that larger quantities and more varied types of fresh food products are available. These and other factors have contributed to populations which are fitter and live longer than before, so that quality of life rather than mere survival has become all-important.

With these increased expectations of health, however, has come a degree of dissatisfaction with conventional medicine, particularly in the field of obstetrics, when women are generally well and want to do all that they can for their babies. Developments in contraception, infertility treatment, genetics and more sophisticated obstetric technology have enabled many grateful women to plan and space their pregnancies, with reduced perinatal, infant and maternal mortality and morbidity statistics across Europe and the USA. On the other hand, some consumers have sought to redress the balance of power between themselves and the medical profession. Many women have resisted the mechanization of pregnancy and birth and wish to regain autonomy in decision making, focusing on childbirth as a normal physiological life event, unlike obstetricians who regard it as potentially pathological and only normal in retrospect.

In Britain this has led to calls for more natural births, with more facilities for home births. Fragmentation of maternity care and consumer and carer dissatisfaction eventually led to the Government review which produced the 'Changing Childbirth' report,[1] which advocates 'choice, control and continuity' for women. Midwives and obstetricians have been forced to examine their working practices and to make them more woman-centred, offering a flexible, accessible and approachable service within current economic constraints. In other European countries, notably the Netherlands, the status of midwives has always been good, with many countries, such as France and Germany, acknowledging midwifery as a profession separate from nursing and with childbirth being seen, as far as possible, as a non-medical event.

In the USA, one could argue that parental dissatisfaction has fuelled the litigation process in obstetrics, as one of the few ways in which the consumer can retaliate against a medical establishment which seeks to control their every move. In some states women have, until recently, been forced to seek help from lay midwives, sometimes practising illegally, in order to acquire individualized, holistic, woman-centred care. However, the status of independently practising certified nurse-midwives is currently being re-examined as the demand for high quality, accessible and cost-effective care grows apace and some states are accrediting these professionals for the first time.[2] In Canada, the midwifery profession was eventually legalized in 1993, after years of campaigning by both midwives and mothers. This return to midwifery-led care across the Western world has assisted the empowerment of women and restored 'control' to its rightful owners – the mothers themselves.

Homeopathy in maternity care

Complementary therapies are seen to offer additional choices to women during pregnancy and childbirth. They are gentler and usually safer than pharmaceutical drugs with their associated side-effects. The holistic philosophy of complementary medicine takes into account not only the physical state of the woman but also her emotional, psychological and spiritual well-being. Unlike much of orthodox medicine which often denigrates the opinions of the woman and ignores small verbal and non-verbal clues which she gives, complementary medicine takes all of these into account in order to obtain as full a picture as possible of the woman's health.

Homeopathy offers a gentle system of medicine which is particularly suited to use for pregnant and childbearing women, at a time when many other drugs are contraindicated. The minute doses used in homeopathic remedies have been tested on healthy volunteers in low doses and found to be totally safe for both the mother and the fetus and, when used appropriately, without producing unwanted side-effects. Whereas extended use of certain pharmaceutical drugs can eventually lead to resistance, allergies and ultimately a breakdown in the immune system, homeopathy can aid the body's energy and trigger the person's innate capabilities for self-healing. It can be useful in relieving the physiological disorders of pregnancy, labour and the puerperium and in the neonate, but can also be used to treat complications, either alone or in conjunction with conventional treatments.

Across the Westernized world, homeopathic medicines are readily available 'over the counter' but, as with any remedies, they must be treated with respect. Using homeopathy requires one to alter the traditional way in which most people view medicines. Unlike conventional pharmaceutical preparations, it is not appropriate to offer one set remedy for a condition which orthodox medicine has given a specific label, a situation which Roy[3] likens to fitting together a jigsaw puzzle to complete the correct picture. For example, the symptom of nausea and vomiting in pregnancy may take many forms – nausea alone, minimal vomiting, profuse vomiting – any of which may or may not be associated with food, aromas, tiredness, anxiety, gestation or other conditions. The homeopath therefore would seek to discover the exact nature of the symptom of nausea and vomiting, together with the factors which make it better or worse and the person's related emotions, before matching the entire symptom picture to the most appropriate remedy. Midwives and others involved in conventional maternity care have much to learn from homeopathy's system of diagnosis, even if they do not wish or are not able to offer the remedies to their clients.

In Britain, homeopathy ranks among the top five complementary therapies,[4] is available on the National Health Service and is tacitly approved by the medical profession, some of whom use the therapy alongside conventional practice. In Europe, homeopathy is favoured as an adjunct to orthodox medicine, particularly in Germany, France, the Netherlands and Scandinavia. The European Community's 1992 homeopathy directive makes it mandatory for member states to set up a system of registration for homeopathic products or to accept the decision of other member states, to facilitate the free importation and sale of the remedies across the Community. In the United States, homeopathic remedies are recognized as drugs by the Federal Drug Agency, with approximately 95% being available over the counter, and homeopathy is acknowledged as a legitimate medical practice and is incorporated into the training of doctors in many medical schools. American medical practitioners and osteopaths use homeopathy, as well as nurse practitioners, physician assistants, dentists, chiropractors and acupuncturists.

There are several ways by which midwives, maternity nurses and medical practitioners may come into contact with homeopathy. Interest may be expressed by the mother herself, as she may have used the remedies before conception or wish to use them if necessary during her pregnancy and labour. Some women may arrive in the delivery suite with packets of various homeopathic remedies for use in labour. Occasionally a mother may be accompanied by a registered homeopath whom she wishes to assist her during the birth. Alternatively maternity care staff may have an interest in or be qualified in homeopathy; for example, the family medical practitioner may combine allopathic and complementary medicine or an individual midwife within a maternity unit may also be trained to use homeopathy. In many respects it may be beneficial to the mother for the roles of midwife and homeopath to be combined in the one person, to avoid fragmentation of care and the potential for misinterpretation or lack of communication which can occur when two professionals with different philosophies and priorities are involved in caring for the same woman. Where a visiting homeopath attends a woman who is receiving conventional maternity care, every effort should be made by all the professionals involved to communicate adequately in order to provide optimum care for the mother.

However, midwifery and medical staff must always remember the mother's right to administer substances such as homeopathic remedies to herself and be careful not to override these rights or appear judgemental.[5,6] It is much better if the mother feels able to share with her carers the fact that she is using homeopathic remedies rather than concealing it in the belief that staff will disapprove. Facilitating communication and collaboration with the parents, rather than initiating confrontation and conflict with them, will result in greater cooperation from the mother, whilst enabling maternity staff to provide the most appropriate care.

The possibility of midwives using homeopathic remedies within their practice will depend on a variety of factors. In Britain, the United Kingdom Central Council facilitates the development of additional skills and the acquisition of new knowledge to enhance practice. However, midwives must be able to demonstrate that they are adequately and appropriately trained to administer the remedies. They must also work within department protocols laid down by midwifery and/or medical management and should clearly differentiate their roles as midwife and homeopath.[5,7,8]

In some respects, midwives in Britain and Europe are in a better position to explore the incorporation of complementary therapies into their work than their American counterparts. The profession of midwifery is identified separately from that of nursing; many midwives have undertaken education programmes specifically to prepare them to work as midwives, without having first qualified as nurses. Midwives generally have greater autonomy in Europe than in America, although this situation is changing as more nurse-midwives become eligible to practise. In those American states which accredit independently practising certified nurse-midwives, the incorporation of homeopathy may be facilitated. In many European countries the midwife may be the first and only health professional consulted by a woman for

the duration of the child-bearing experience and the status of the midwife is on a par with medical colleagues. It is recognized that the midwife is the expert in normal childbirth while the obstetrician is the expert in abnormal obstetrics.

However, whatever the current status of midwives and maternity nurses, all practitioners almost universally offer advice and information to mothers and their families and may be able to provide guidance about the appropriate use of homeopathy during pregnancy and childbirth. Obviously this information must be accurate, based on sound, contemporary, research-based (where possible) knowledge and must not contravene any regulations laid down locally.

One of the commonest questions which mothers ask regarding the use of homeopathy is about the universal remedy arnica, which is excellent for relieving bruising, trauma and shock.[9] It could conceivably be available in every delivery suite and postnatal ward in the Westernized world, for it is inexpensive and highly effective. However, midwives would be acting outside the limits of their practice if they suggested its use to a woman without being able to give her sufficient information to make her own decision about it.

Research-based practice

As with any other midwifery practice, the use of homeopathy must be based on currently available research findings. Research into homeopathy is somewhat limited, although increasing, but the therapy is unlikely to be accepted fully by the medical establishment until more scientific evidence is forthcoming. Gibson et al[10] showed a significant improvement in rheumatoid arthritic patients who used homeopathy and similar results were demonstrated in those with osteoarthritis.[11] Kleijnen et al[12] undertook a review of 107 trials of homeopathy and questioned their validity. Taylor-Reilly[13] explored the use of homeopathic remedies in the treatment of asthma and hayfever, although again sceptics queried both the methodology and the results. Taylor-Reilly and Taylor[14] had themselves written of the difficulties involved in undertaking research into homeopathy, highlighting the problem of using randomized double-blind controlled trials to investigate a system of medicine which depends so particularly on individualizing treatment.

Double-blind studies have, however, been carried out, including Brigo and Serpelloni's 1991 study of 60 cases of migraine[15] and Carey's 1986 comparison of Borax and Candida homeopathic remedies for the treatment of vaginal discharge.[16] Jacobs et al[17,18] explored the use of homeopathy to treat childhood diarrhoea in Nicaragua. Trials have also been undertaken in the field of dentistry[19] and veterinary work.[20]

There appears to be little homeopathy research specifically related to human obstetrics, although two trials are currently being completed.[21] Caulophyllum has been shown to shorten the average length of labour and reduce pain and the risk of complications.[22–25] The dearth of related research is disappointing, considering the benefits to be gained by pregnant women from using homeopathic medicines, but until more studies have been undertaken many orthodox medical practitioners are unlikely to accept homeopathy without reservations.

Homeopathy can, however, be used safely by appropriately informed midwives for, in homeopathic terms, pregnancy, labour and the puerperium are classed as acute conditions. Chronic conditions require consultation with a fully qualified homeopath to ascertain the correct constitutional remedies whereas, in many maternity situations, universal remedies can be effective. Used correctly, homeopathic medicines will treat physiological and pathological problems during the child-bearing phase, without side-effects. It must be stressed, however, that midwives are responsible for caring for women with normal pregnancies, labours and puerperia and must acknowledge the boundaries of their practice according to the country in which they are working.

This book, written by a homeopath, provides midwives and maternity nurses with an overview of the potential for using homeopathy for pregnant and child-bearing women and their babies. It is not intended that midwives should use it to replace a thorough training in homeopathy, if they wish and are permitted to incorporate the therapy into their practice. However, it does offer a useful source of reference, in an easily read, cross-referencing format, which may be helpful when midwives come into contact with homeopaths or with mothers wishing to use the remedies on their own responsibility. As more courses specifically relating homeopathic principles to maternity care become available, it will serve as a valuable textbook for students and later for qualified midwives and homeopaths. I am pleased to support this book at a time when the use of complementary therapies within maternity care is slowly becoming more acceptable.

REFERENCES

1. Department of Health 1993 Changing childbirth – report of the Expert Maternity Group. HMSO, London
2. Williams D 1994 Credentialling certified nurse-midwives. Journal of Nurse-Midwifery 39(4): 258–264
3. Roy M 1994 The principles of homoeopathic philosophy: a self-directed learning text. Churchill Livingstone, London
4. British Medical Association 1993 Complementary medicine – new approaches to good practice. Oxford University Press, Oxford
5. UKCC 1994 Midwife's code of practice. UKCC, London
6. UKCC 1996 Guidelines for professional practice. UKCC, London
7. UKCC 1992 The scope of professional practice. UKCC, London
8. Tiran D 1996 Aromatherapy in midwifery practice. Baillière Tindall, London
9. Hofmeyr G J, Piccioni V, Blauhof P 1990 Postpartum homoeopathic Arnica Montana: a potency finding pilot study. British Journal of Clinical Practice 44: 619–621
10. Gibson R G, Gibson S L M, MacNeill D A, Watson-Buchanan W 1980 Homoeopathic therapy in rheumatoid arthritis: evaluation by double-blind clinical trial. British Journal of Clinical Pharmacology 9: 453–459
11. Shipley M, Berry H, Broster G, Jenkins M, Clover A, William I 1983 Controlled trial of homoeopathic treatment of osteoarthritis. Lancet 1: 97–98
12. Kleijnen J, Knipschild P, ter Riet G 1991 Clinical trials of homoeopathy. British Medical Journal 302: 316–323
13. Taylor-Reilly D 1992 Hay fever and asthma trials. Homoeopathy Today 12(8): 12–14
14. Taylor-Reilly D, Taylor M A 1988 The difficulty with homoeopathy: a brief review of principles, methods and research. Complementary Medical Research 3(1): 70–78
15. Brigo B, Serpelloni G 1991 Homoeopathic treatment of migraine: a randomised double-blind controlled study of 60 cases (homoeopathy v placebo). Berlin Journal of Research and Homoeopathy 1: 98–106
16. Carey H 1986 Double-blind clinical trial of Borax and Candida in the treatment of vaginal discharge. Committee of the British Homoeopathy Research Group 15: 12–14
17. Jacobs J, Jimenez L M, Gloyd S, Crothers D, Casares F, Gaitan M 1993 Treatment of acute childhood diarrhoea with homoeopathic medicine: a randomized clinical trial in Nicaragua. British Homoeopathic Journal 82: 83–86
18. Jacobs J, Jimenez L M, Gloyd S, Gale J, Crothers D 1994 Treatment of acute childhood diarrhoea with homoeopathic medicine: a randomized clinical trial in Nicaragua. Pediatrics 93: 719–725
19. Pinsent R J, Baker G P, Ives G et al (1986) Does Arnica reduce pain and bleeding after dental extraction? Committee of the British Homoeopathy Research Group 15: 3–11
20. Day C E 1984 Control of stillbirth in pigs using homoeopathy. Veterinary Record 114: 216
21. Webb P 1992 Homoeopathy for midwives (and pregnant women). British Homoeopathic Association, London
22. Arnal-Laserre M N 1986 Preparation a l'accouchement par homeopathie: experimentation en double insu versus placebo (dissertation). Academie de Paris, Universite Rene Descartes
23. Coudert-Deguillaume M 1981 Etude experimentale de l'action du Caulophyllim dans la faux travail et la dystocie de demarrage (dissertation). Universite de Limoges, Limoges
24. Dorfman P et al 1987 Preparation for childbirth by homoeopathy. Cahiers de Biotherapie 94: 77–81
25. Ventoskovskij H M, Popov A V 1990 Homoeopathy as a practical alternative to traditional obstetric methods. British Homoeopathic Journal 79: 201–205

A brief homeopathic 1.2
history

Throughout medical history there have been two basic schools of thought – one treating disease with 'opposites' and the other treating with 'similars'. For example, the first school would treat constipation with laxatives, which produce diarrhoea in a healthy person; the second would treat it using a substance known to cause constipation. The 18th-century German doctor Samuel Hahnemann founded and developed the system of homeopathy, meaning 'similar suffering', on this second principle, which may be traced back to the ancient Greeks and the doctor and philosopher Hippocrates and probably originates with the ancient Egyptians. In more recent times, the idea was pursued by the 16th-century Swiss healer and philosopher Paracelsus, but it was Hahnemann who developed an entire system of healing on the principle *similia similibus curentur* or 'let like be cured with like'.

Samuel Hahnemann (1755–1843) had become increasingly disillusioned with the cruel and ineffective medical treatments of his time (blood-letting, purging, poisonous drugs with terrible side-effects) and gave up his practice in order to concentrate on study, research, writing and translation. While translating Dr William Cullen's *A Treatise on Materia Medica* in 1789, Hahnemann found himself disputing the author's theory that the substance Cinchona cures malaria because of its bitterness. He embarked on an experiment, taking the substance himself, and came to the conclusion that Cinchona was effective because of its ability to induce malaria symptoms, i.e. periodic fever, sweating and palpitations, in a healthy individual.

Further experiments followed which confirmed the principle of similars. The testing procedure, still in use today, found the healing properties of any substance by observing the symptoms it produced in a healthy volunteer. This procedure is called a *proving*. The symptoms of accidental poisonings were also observed and after several years of gathering material, Hahnemann returned to medical practice using a homeopathic basis for his prescriptions. Patients were prescribed a remedy whose 'symptom picture', based on provings, best matched that of their symptoms.

His results verified his theory, but using his medicines in crude form produced undesirable effects. He experimented with smaller and smaller doses and then began to dilute the medicines. This created a new problem, because the diluted medicines no longer effected a cure. Vigorous shaking or *succussion* was introduced, with the result that the 'potentized remedy' not only lacked undesirable effects, but had somehow become more effective. He concluded that dilution and succussion had together released the strength or energy of the substance and dissipated its toxic effects. Undeterred by the fact that this phenomenon could not be fully explained, then as now (see Research section, p. 9), Hahnemann spent the rest of his life documenting his findings and developing the philosophy and practical methodology behind his system of medicine.

In 1811 and 1821 he published his *Materia Medica Pura*, representing the results of his provings. In 1828 came *Chronic Diseases and Their Homoeopathic Cure*. The sixth edition of his *Organon of Medicine*, published after his death, in which the philosophy and rules of homeopathy are set out, remains the inspiration and guide of successive generations of homeopaths. However, it was not until after the central European cholera epidemic of 1831, when those treated with homeopathy had a far higher recovery rate than those under the care of orthodox physicians, that homeopathy made a really significant impact. By the time of Hahnemann's death, homeopathy had attracted enough medically trained and influential followers for it to spread to several other countries.

Constantine Hering (1800–1880), who had originally been asked to disprove homeopathy during his medical studies at Leipzig University, became actively involved in the homeopathic world after receiving successful treatment for an infected wound. In 1827 he travelled to South America where he carried out his now famous provings of the bushmaster snake venom Lachesis. On his way back to Europe he stopped off in Philadelphia where he stayed to become the intellectual leader of 19th-century homeopathy in the USA. Throughout his life Hering proved many substances, wrote extensively, expanding Hahnemann's theories, and is best remembered for his Laws of Cure.[1]

HOMEOPATHY IN THE USA

Homeopathy was readily accepted in America shortly after Dutch homeopath Hans Gram emigrated there in 1825. The spread was so rapid that the homeopaths established America's first national medical society, the American Institute of Homeopathy, in 1844. The rival American Medical Association was set up 2 years later, discouraging its members from having anything to do with homeopathy. However, homeopathy survived the various attempts to destroy it and public demand for it grew, reaching a peak in the period 1860–1890 when news of its successes in treating infectious epidemic diseases such as the Cincinnati cholera epidemic of 1849 and the southern yellow fever epidemic of 1878 became widely known. Training establishments, hospitals, mental asylums and sanatoria were numerous and flourished.

Homeopathy was particularly popular with followers of Swedenborg (1689–1772), a Swedish theologian and philosopher, whose writings were studied by those concerned with the conflict between religion and Darwinism. The American physician James Tyler Kent (1849–1916) was a follower of Swedenborg and he turned his energies to homeopathy after his wife was successfully treated by a homeopath. Kent's *Philosophy* and *Materia Medica* and particularly his *Repertory* are still among the most widely used homeopathic texts. His use of the higher potency remedies (at that time from 30 and above; see Potency section, p. 12) was eventually to lead to a split among homeopaths in the USA, with the 'purists' being the high potency prescribers, basing their prescription on a total symptom picture following the ideas of Kent, and the 'revolutionists' being the low potency (up to 30) prescribers, basing their remedy selection on the pathological diagnosis alone. This division, together with the developments in orthodox medicine, the rise of the pharmaceutical industry and the closure of many homeopathic teaching institutions in 1911, eventually took its toll on the American homeopathic establishment and by 1918 only seven homeopathic hospitals remained. However, recent years have seen homeopathy becoming more popular again, a trend which can be seen in many other countries where homeopathy is practised.

HOMEOPATHY IN BRITAIN

Britain was introduced to homeopathy when the young doctor Frederick Quin (1799–1878) set up a homeopathic practice in 1832. He was one of a group of Hahnemann's closest colleagues to come to Britain around that time. Other members of the group included Dr Paul Curie (1799–1853), the silk merchant Mr William Leaf (1790–1873) and the Reverend Thomas Rapoul Everest (1801–1873)[2] but Dr Quin separated from this group in order to concentrate on introducing homeopathy to the medically qualified. In 1844 he founded the British Homoeopathic Society and 5 years later, the London Homoeopathic Hospital. Quin had many rich and powerful friends, among them Sir Henry Tyler (1827–1908), father of the influential homeopathic doctor Margaret Tyler (1857–1943) who trained under Dr James Tyler Kent in Chicago. Sir Henry later set up a trust, known as the Henry Tyler Scholarship, to enable young doctors to study homeopathy in the USA.[2] Other influential friends included members of the House of Lords and it was this which saved homeopathy from being outlawed by a medical bill introduced to Parliament after the Crimean War. Homeopathy grew in popularity and throughout the late 19th and early 20th centuries further homeopathic hospitals were opened in Bristol, Glasgow, Tunbridge Wells and Liverpool. In London during the period around 1880–1900, an informal gathering of several leading homeopathic doctors known as the Cooper Club would meet regularly to exchange notes and experiences. The club members were chiefly Dr Robert Cooper (1844–1903), Dr Thomas Skinner (1825–1906) and Dr James Compton Burnett (1840–1901), who were later joined by Dr John Henry Clarke (1853–1931).[2] Clarke became very well-known, but the hostile reaction to homeopathy among his orthodox colleagues prompted him to leave the British Homoeopathic Society and channel his energy into teaching homeopathy to laypersons. Among his pupils were Noel Puddephatt (1899–1978) whose own pupils include the well-known homeopaths Phyllis Speight, Sheilagh Creasy and George Vithoulkas. Other important homeopathic teachers included Thomas Maughan (1902–1976) and John da Monte (1916–1975), whose pupils formed the Society of Homoeopaths in 1977.[2]

Although homeopathy had gone into a lengthy period of obscurity it was included as an approved method of treatment when the National Health Service was established in 1948. This enabled the homeopathic hospitals to provide homeopathic treatment under the National Health Service. As demand for homeopathy has again grown over recent years an increasing number of general practitioner surgeries have made homeopathic treatment available to their patients. As the number of professional homeopaths who have not undergone orthodox medical training is also increasing and they are being acknowledged as professionals in their own right, they too are becoming an accepted part of the National Health Service in much the same way as the chiropractors and osteopaths. An increasing number now work as consultants to general practitioners, although the majority still work in private clinics working on a referral basis.

Today, homeopathy is recognized and practised in many countries in varying degrees. It has also evolved differently in different countries.

Research into homeopathy

Many sceptics allege that homeopathy is nothing but the administration of a placebo, saying that the small doses used cannot possibly have the effects attributed to them. The argument for homeopathy is also not helped by the apparent inability of current scientific theories to explain the mechanism behind the action of homeopathic remedies. There is, however, some compelling clinical and laboratory research evidence available to suggest that homeopathic remedies do indeed work.

CLINICAL RESEARCH

In 1991, three non-homeopath professors of medicine carried out a review or *meta-analysis* of 25 years of clinical studies using homeopathic medicines, in order to evaluate the overall results of the experiments.[3] Out of the 107 controlled trials reviewed, 81 showed that homeopathic

remedies were effective, 24 showed they were ineffective and two were inconclusive. Out of all the studies, the researchers found only 22 whose methodology was not flawed in some way, owing to the fact that they had been carried out primarily by clinicians inadequately trained in research methods. Of these, 15 showed that homeopathic remedies were effective and the researchers concluded that the review would 'probably be sufficient for establishing homeopathy as a regular treatment for certain conditions'.

More recent studies include clinical trials evaluating homeopathy in the treatment of asthma.[4] In this study the researchers first discovered which substances 24 asthma sufferers were allergic to, then randomized the subjects into treatment and placebo groups. Those chosen for treatment were given the substance to which they were most allergic in the form of homeopathic potency 30C. (Usually remedies are prescribed on a person's individual symptoms.) The researchers gave the name *homeopathic immunotherapy* to their means of individualizing the remedy.

The subjects were then evaluated by both homeopathic and conventional physicians and the results showed that 82% of those given the homeopathic remedy had improved as opposed to 38% of those in the placebo group. The researchers then carried out a meta-analysis reviewing the data from three studies performed on allergic conditions, bringing the total number of subjects to 202. The results followed a similar pattern, leading to the conclusion that homeopathy was effective.

Another recent study involved a randomized double-blind, placebo-controlled study of 81 children suffering from diarrhoea.[5] This also gave positive results, with children treated with an individually chosen remedy recovering 20% faster than those given placebo.

A study involving individualized homeopathic care was carried out in the treatment of rheumatoid arthritis.[6] This again gave positive results, with 82% of those receiving the homeopathic remedy experiencing relief while 21% of the placebo group experienced similar relief.

Another study which gave positive results was the double-blind, placebo controlled crossover trial into the effect of homeopathic treatment on fibrositis.[7] This time the subjects selected fitted the symptoms of the remedy Rhus tox.

In 1990, clinical studies of the effect of the homeopathic remedy Caulophyllum in normal labour were carried out in Italy,[8] to verify its applicability and investigate its toxicity during labour. (Caulophyllum is often used to establish effective contractions in labour and encourage cervical dilatation – see Suggested Uses for Caulophyllum in the Materia Medica section, p. 112). Twenty-two healthy primigravidae who had gone into labour spontaneously at term were given 50 mg of sucrose-lactose granules impregnated with Caulophyllum 7C. The dose of 5 granules per hour, repeated for a maximum of 4 hours, was given during the active phase of labour and the effects were noted and evaluated during phase 1 of the study.

In phase 2, the 17 women from the original group who had normal and spontaneous labour and parturition were compared to a random control group of 34 women, selected on the same criteria of eligibility as the original Caulophyllum group. The differences between these two groups were then evaluated. The results showed that the remedy was well tolerated and did not produce adverse reactions in either mother or fetus. The Caulophyllum-treated women showed an improvement in emotional state during treatment, especially if they belonged to a further subgroup who were introverted in character and had a history of dysmenorrhoea. The duration of labour was reduced by about 90 minutes.

Clinical trials have also been carried out on animals, which are not suggestible and therefore not prone to the placebo effect. The homeopathic remedy Caulophyllum 30C was tried on pigs, to see if it could lower the rate of stillbirths.[9] The placebo group had 20.8% stillbirths, while the remedy group had fewer, at 10.3%, giving positive results.

LABORATORY TRIALS

By assessing changes in cells, tissues, organs, enzymes, viruses, etc., these trials are able to show biological activity of homeopathic remedies that cannot be explained as a placebo response and are also capable of providing more clues to how remedies work.

Investigations to provide evidence for the infinitesimal dose have been carried out in the areas of biochemistry, botany, bacteriology and zoology. Well-known examples include the experiments carried out by Boyd in 1941 showing that microdoses of mercuric chloride had statistically significant effects on the diastase activity of germinating seeds[10] and the work of Benveniste who tested highly diluted doses of an antibody on basophils.[11] This caused great controversy after the prestigious journal *Nature* published the study and later disputed the findings, which led to the theory that water molecules retained 'memory' of a substance even when there was little chance of a single molecule of the original substance remaining.

Despite all the positive evidence as to the efficacy of homeopathy to date, it is unlikely to become generally accepted by the medical profession and public until science can clearly demonstrate how it works. Perhaps the quantum physicists hold the key to the solution, but until the answer is found, the results of clinical research will always be questioned because of the difficulty in reconciling the individual nature of homeopathic treatment with the rigorous standardization requirements of modern clinical research.

REFERENCES

1. Hering C 1865 Hahnemann's three rules concerning the rank of symptoms. Hahnemannian Monthly 1: 5–12
2. Morell P 1995 A brief history of British lay homoeopathy (based upon a paper given at the 1st international conference on the history of homoeopathy at the Robert Bosch Institute for the History of Medicine in Stuttgart, 4–6 April 1995). Journal of the Society of Homoeopaths 59: 471–475
3. Kleijnen J, Knipschild P, ter Reit G 1991 Clinical trials of homoeopathy. British Medical Journal 302: 316–323
4. Reilly D, Taylor M, Beattie N et al 1994 Is evidence for homoeopathy reproducible? Lancet 344: 1601–1606
5. Jacobs J, Jimenez L M, Gloyd S S, Gale J, Crothers D 1994 Treatment of acute childhood diarrhoea with homoeopathic medicine: a randomized clinical trial in Nicaragua. Pediatrics 93: 719–725
6. Gibson R G, Gibson S, MacNeill A D, Watson-Buchanan W 1980 Homoeopathic therapy in rheumatoid arthritis: evaluation by double-blind clinical therapeutic trial. British Journal of Clinical Pharmacology 9: 453–459
7. Fisher P, Greenwood A, Huskisson E C, Turner P, Belon P 1989 Effect of homoeopathic treatment on fibrositis (primary fibromyalgia). British Medical Journal 299: 365–366.
8. Eid P, Felisi E, Sideri M 1993 Applicability of homoeopathic *caulophyllum thalicroides* during labour. British Homoeopathic Journal 82: 245
9. Day C 1986 Control of stillbirth in pigs using homeopathy. Journal of the American Institute of Homeopathy 779(4): 146–147
10. Boyd W E 1941 The action of microdoses of mercuric chloride on diastase. British Homoeopathic Journal 31: 1–18 and 32: 106–111
11. Benveniste J, Davenas E, Amara J et al 1988 Human basophil degranulation triggered by very dilute antiserum against IgE. Nature 333: 816–818

FURTHER READING

Bellavite P, Signorini A 1995 Homeopathy: a frontier in medical science. North Atlantic Books, Berkeley, California
Coulter H L 1980 Homeopathic science and modern medicine – the physics of healing with microdoses. North Atlantic Books, Berkeley, California
Coulter H L 1995 Divided legacy. North Atlantic Books, Berkeley, California
Danciger E 1987 The emergence of homoeopathy – alchemy into medicine. Century, London
Ullman D 1989 Homeopathy – medicine for the 21st century. Thorsons, Wellingborough
Ullman D 1995 The consumer's guide to homeopathy: the definitive resource for understanding homeopathic medicine and making it work for you. G P Putnam's Sons, New York

Homeopathic remedies 1.3

Remedies come from many sources and the 'common' name of a remedy will usually reveal its origins. Sources include:

- plants, e.g. Arnica (*Arnica montana*, Leopard's bane or mountain tobacco);
- vegetables, e.g. Allium cepa (*Allium cepa*, red onion);
- minerals – elements, e.g. Sulphur ('flowers' of sulphur, S), and compounds, e.g. Natrum muriaticum (sodium chloride, NaCl, common salt);
- organic substances, e.g. Petroleum (rock oil);
- chemicals, e.g. Sulphuricum acidum (sulphuric acid, H_2SO_4);
- animals, insects, e.g. Apis (*Apis mellifica*, honey bee);
- disease products (producing a type of remedy known as a *nosode*), e.g. Tuberculinum bovinum (tubercular preparation made from infected lymph glands of cattle);
- healthy glands and glandular secretions (producing a type of remedy known as a *sarcode*), e.g. Thyroidinum (made from the dried thyroid gland of the sheep);
- conventional drugs, e.g. Naprosyn (made from the non-steroid anti-inflammatory drug of the same name).

How remedies are made[1]

Remedies are available in a number of so-called 'potencies', e.g. 6X, 6C, which refers to their method of preparation.

The initial preparation of a remedy varies according to the substance, but the general method of preparation (known as *potentization*) of each remedy is similar, involving repeated processes of dilution and violent shaking (known as *succussion*). For example, Arnica 6C denotes:

Source material:	Arnica
Number of repeated dilution and succussion processes:	6
Dilution scale (1:100):	Centisimal

In the case of a plant remedy, a 'mother tincture' is first made by dissolving the substance in an alcohol and water solution. Next, depending on whether a decimal (X) or centesimal (C) potency is to be made, one drop of mother tincture is added to either 9 or 99 drops of alcohol and water solution respectively. The resulting dilution is then succussed 100 times. The first potency on the chosen scale (i.e. 1X or 1C) has now been made.

To make the second potency, one drop of the first potency is added to either 9 or 99 drops of fresh solvent and then succussed 100 times. This process is repeated to make the next potency and so on. The higher the number on a remedy, the greater its potency.

Potency

Homeopathic remedies can be made to any desired potency by simply repeating the dilution and succussion process the required number of times. A number of 'standard' potencies are available, the most readily accessible in Britain being the 6C and 30C.

The higher the potency, the more carefully it must be prescribed, as its clinical action will be stronger and of longer duration. As a 'rule of thumb' the lower potencies (6X and 6C) are used for minor physical complaints of an acute nature, as their action is mainly concentrated on the physical level of being. The 30th potency has greater dynamic strength and therefore a deeper physical and mental/emotional action. It is the 30C potency which the midwife will find most helpful, as it is used for symptoms requiring immediate attention and accompanied by great pain.

Higher potencies, such as the 200C, 1M (the 'M' denoting 1000 potency) and higher, act more deeply and should be treated with the utmost respect. They should only be used in consultation with a professional homeopath who has come to know the mother well during in-depth consultations.

Remedy availability

Although many standard 6C homeopathic remedies are now readily available in health food shops and High Street chemists in Britain, it is worthwhile obtaining remedies directly from a specialist homeopathic pharmacy. Not only do these provide the widest range of potencies, correctly packed, stored and supplied to prolong shelf-life and prevent contamination, they are also able to make up non-standard remedy forms and potencies on request (see Useful Addresses section – Homeopathic Pharmacies, p. 148).

Homeopathic remedies are most commonly available in hard tablet form because saccharum lactose ('sac lac' or sugar of cow's milk), from which the tablets are made, has been found to be the ideal carrier medium for the potentized remedy. Non-standard variants include soft tablets, globules, sucrose, powders, wafers and liquid potencies.

HARD TABLETS

The standard form of tablets, which dissolve slowly and need to be held in the mouth. May be given in crushed form.

SOFT TABLETS

Dissolve quickly and easily under the tongue and do not need to be chewed. For this reason they are particularly useful during labour. Once crushed, they are ideal for babies. Recommended for labour kits.

GLOBULES

Tiny poppy seed-sized pills. A few grains are dissolved in the mouth.

SUCROSE OR SUGAR DRAGEES

Small, round sugar balls made from sucrose available in a variety of sizes. The smallest resemble globules and are frequently used when making up a pocket travel kit.

POWDERS

Wrapped individually in small squares of paper. The powder is either dissolved under the tongue or added to a small amount of water and held in the mouth for a few seconds before swallowing.

WAFERS

Individually wrapped rice paper wafers used for people sensitive to both milk and sugar.

LIQUID POTENCIES

Supplied in dropper bottles. The dose is administered either neat on the tongue or diluted in water, in which case 5 drops are added to a small amount of water and held in the mouth for a few seconds before swallowing. Used for people allergic to cow's milk. Ideal for babies.

Storage of remedies

Remedies should be stored in their well-stoppered original container in a cool, dark, dry place, well away from strong-smelling substances such as perfumes, cough mixtures, mothballs, aromatherapy peppermint oil and eucalyptus oil, Tiger Balm, Vicks or Olbas Oil. Empty containers should not be reused.

Correctly stored, the remedies will keep their strength for many years without deteriorating.

How remedies are administered

It is preferable not to eat, smoke, brush the teeth or drink anything except water at least 10–15 minutes before or after taking a remedy to prevent contamination and ensure optimum remedy action.

Tablets, powders, sucrose, globules and wafers should be dissolved under the tongue, where they are absorbed into the bloodstream. Liquid potencies can be dropped on to the tongue directly or diluted with a little water and held in the mouth for a few seconds before swallowing.

The remedy should only be touched by the person actually taking it. Therefore any tablets that have fallen on to the floor or that have been given out and not used must be thrown away. For an adult, one tablet is first tipped into the lid of the remedy bottle and then on to the palm of the person taking the remedy. The lid of the bottle is then replaced tightly.

For a baby the tablet is usually crushed between two sterilized plastic spoons (to avoid problems in case of metal allergy) and the powder tipped dry on to the tongue. If this is not possible a little water can be added to the crushed powder on the spoon and then dropped into the mouth. Alternatively the tablet may be dissolved in a clean glass, half filled with water, stirring vigorously each time before giving as needed, a spoonful at a time. The glass or spoon should then be sterilized with boiling water. Liquid potencies can be dropped into the mouth of the infant directly or after diluting with a little water.

It is worthwhile noting that *it is the number of times the remedy is repeated which increases its effect, not the size of the single dose*. Therefore, the physical size of the tablet or the precise quantity of water added when dissolving a remedy are not of great importance (see Homeopathic Principles and Prescribing – Provings, p. 16).

REFERENCES

1. Kunzli J 1982 Organon of medicine, Samuel Hahnemann: a new translation. Gollancz, London, paragraphs 264–271

FURTHER READING

Boyd H 1981 Introduction to homoeopathic medicine. Beaconsfield, Beaconsfield, Bucks
Creasy S 1995 Notes on the nosodes *Tuberculinum* and *Bacillinum*. SCHB (Publishing), London
Crockett P 1995 The unfolded organon – a precis of Hahnemann's sixth edition. Islington Centre of Homoeopathy, London
Koehler G 1986 The handbook of homoeopathy – its principles and practice. Thorsons, Wellingborough
Vithoulkas G 1986 The science of homeopathy. Thorsons, Wellingborough

Homeopathic principles and prescribing

The principles of homeopathy as laid down by Samuel Hahnemann in *The Organon of Medicine* are crucial to successful prescribing and are outlined below to provide an insight into how homeopaths are trained to think and practise.

The principles can be divided into two categories, i.e. those which apply to the human being and those which apply to the cure of disease.

The human being

In homeopathy it is acknowledged that a human being is not merely a collection of physical parts, but that there are other non-physical parts which are also of great importance. The following principles are used to gain an understanding of the patient.

THE VITAL FORCE[1]

This term was used by Hahnemann to describe the balancing mechanism that keeps us in health, that gives us life and is absent at our death.

The human being is a dynamis whose well-being is governed by its inner nature – the dynamic, spiritual and vital force. The physical body is merely the outer manifestation of an inner energetic state. If the vital force is in a state of well-being the person is in a state of health on all planes of existence. If the condition of this force is altered by overwhelming influences of any kind, changes will occur which are manifested as symptoms. These are expressions of the un-ease of the vital force and the person has 'disease'. Since the whole person is a manifestation of their innermost energetic condition, a return to health can only be brought about by restoring a state of well-being to the vital force through change in this energetic condition. This can be achieved by the energetic stimulus provided via the correctly selected homeopathic remedy.

SUSCEPTIBILITY[2]

This term refers to the state of the vital force and its ability to adapt to new conditions and was adopted by Hahnemann to explain why stresses do not produce a specific disease in the whole population at the same time and also why individuals are not ill all the time.

A stress of any kind cannot alter a person's state of health unconditionally. It does so only when the person's organism is sufficiently disposed and susceptible to that particular stress. In this case the person will produce symptoms on which a prescription can be based.

The totality of symptoms[3] or 'cry for help' by the vital force forms the basis for the prescription. The susceptibility and vital force together tell of the energy state of the patient and give an indication of her sensitivity to remedies. Their condition has a bearing on the remedy potency selected.

MIASM[4]

This term, which means 'contamination' or 'deep trouble', was used by Hahnemann to describe a predisposition towards various weaknesses and chronic diseases. Miasms form part of a person's inheritance as they are passed from generation to generation.

Hahnemann formulated his miasm theory during years of experiment and critical observation that certain patients were easily cured with simple remedies or had a natural spontaneous cure while others continually returned with old complaints or new symptoms.[5] All such cases were studied carefully and the obstacles to cure identified as miasms, which he named 'Psora', 'Sycosis' and 'Syphilis'. They can act singly or in combination.

Psora or the 'internal itch' is the fundamental miasm and relates to a general lack of stamina made better by an exciting stimulus. The Sycosis miasm stems from gonorrhoea and relates to excess of any sort – discharges, growths. The Syphilitic miasm stems from syphilis and therefore relates to destruction and degeneration – ulceration, deformity, etc.

An understanding of miasm theory makes 'reading' of the case easier, in terms of symptoms indicating disease patterns, tendencies and possible prognosis.

The cure of disease

The following principles refer to the cure of disease:

THE SIMILIMUM[6]

Anything that produces symptoms of disease in a healthy person can cure a sick person with similar symptoms.

The word 'similar' as opposed to 'identical' is crucial here; for example, the remedy Arsenicum would not automatically be prescribed for a person suffering from arsenic poisoning. The patient's symptom picture, which

could well be that of another remedy, would indicate the true similimum. (Variants on homeopathy which employ 'identicals' are known as isopathy[7] and tautopathy[8] and are not discussed in this book.)

PROVINGS[9]

This is the term given to the process of remedy testing in order to acquire a complete description of the symptoms produced by the substance under investigation.

Hahnemann tested the effects of various substances on himself and other healthy subjects so that a refined picture of symptomatology could be drawn up for prescriptive use. The symptomatology of the remedy could then be matched with that of the patient.

Today homeopaths and their students continue the search for the healing properties of any substance by observing the symptoms it produces when taken repeatedly by a group of healthy volunteers. It has been found that Hahnemann's records are still valid today, as modern provers display symptoms identical to those of the original provers when exposed to the same substance. The results of new provings are published and, in time, incorporated into the standard literature of the Materia Medica[10] and Repertory. Examples of more recent provings include those of chocolate[11] and human breast milk, Lac humanum.[12]

A Materia Medica lists the symptom pictures of each remedy as discovered in the provings, through clinical experience (where symptoms have been helped or cured by a particular remedy in a reasonable number of patients) and through accidental poisoning and toxicology. The many hundreds of remedies are arranged alphabetically and the symptoms of these remedies are arranged according to body area. The professional homeopath works with a number of Materia Medicae compiled by different homeopaths, reflecting their own personal experience and providing a differing amount of detail on each remedy.

A Repertory is a cross-reference for the Materia Medica, being a list of symptoms arranged alphabetically together with the remedy names applying to each symptom. The best known Repertory is that of J T Kent, which remains popular in spite of the publication of more recent repertories such as the *Homoeopathic Medical Repertory* (1993) by Robin Murphy[13] and *Synthesis* (1993) edited by Dr Frederik Schroyens.[14]

POTENCY

This is the result of dilution and succussion (violent shaking) during remedy preparation.

Because the person's innermost energetic condition must be brought back into balance before health of the outer physical body can be restored, the homeopath must not only match the remedy to the patient but select a potency which will cure effectively. To do this, the dynamic stimulus should be just enough to stimulate the vital force of the patient to throw off the disease.[15]

SINGLE REMEDY[16]

Only one remedy should be given at one time. This follows directly from the Law of Similars. Given that we are trying to match the remedy picture with that of the patient, it follows that only one remedy may be used at one time, because two things cannot both be the most similar to another. No provings have been carried out on remedy mixtures.

MINIMUM DOSE[17]

The homeopath seeks to apply the smallest dose possible to nudge the vital force into curative action and to restore its balance. This follows the Arndt–Schultz Law, which states that large doses kill, medium doses inhibit and small doses stimulate.

POSSIBLE ANTIDOTES TO HOMEOPATHIC TREATMENT

In *The Organon of Medicine*, Samuel Hahnemann outlined the substances he believed would counteract the action of a homeopathic remedy.[18] In brief, an antidote can be any stimulus, strong-smelling or deep-acting substance which has a profound effect on the person taking the remedy. Because the remedy acts by stimulating a person's self-healing energy, any stimulus capable of bringing about a significant change in this 'target' energy will cause the remedy to fail. People are therefore sensitive to certain antidotes as well as to certain remedies, e.g. someone who becomes agitated and is unable to sleep at night after drinking coffee is more likely to have their remedy antidoted by it than someone on whom coffee has no effect whatsoever. Although the extent to which this happens is a matter of debate among homeopaths themselves, many advise that the following be avoided during homeopathic treatment as a precautionary measure against possible antidoting:

- coffee
- peppermint
- menthol
- eucalyptus
- camphor.

Because homeopathic remedies provide an energetic, non-chemical stimulus only, they will not interfere with any other medication that may be required during pregnancy, labour, the puerperium and throughout life. The opposite is, however, not always true, as many conventional drugs have a profound action, especially on the physical level, and in effect change the remedy picture so that the previously administered homeopathic remedy becomes inappropriate to the case. If a person already taking prescribed orthodox medication seeks homeopathic help, the homeopathic practitioner must know the effects and side-effects of the drugs in order to evaluate the case correctly, which makes it more difficult to select the correct remedy.

If a woman in labour has chosen to use homeopathy for pain relief and/or for complications and the remedies are proving ineffective it is better to turn to conventional medicine and resume homeopathic treatment during the recovery period. If the homeopathy is proving effective, then it is better to continue with that alone, if possible.

Wherever possible the following should be avoided during homeopathic treatment:

Analgesics
Antacids
Antibiotics
Antifungal foot powders
Antiperspirants
Aromatic massage oils
Aspirin
Bonjela
Camphor
Coffee
Cough/throat lozenges
Cough mixtures
Calpol
Decongestants
Deep Heat
Deodorants
Drops – ear, eye, nose
Eucalyptus
Fisherman's Friend
Karvol capsules
Laxatives
Liniments
Lip salves
Medicated creams
Menthol
Mothballs
Mouthwashes
Oil of cloves
Olbas Oil

Peppermint
Recreational drugs
Tiger Balm
Toothpaste (mint-flavoured)*
Vaporizers
Vicks Vapour Rub
White Horse Oil
Wintergreen
Zinc ointments

Limitations and potential risks of Homeopathy[19]

Homeopathic remedies are generally considered safe but, like all things, they are open to misuse. Repeating a correctly chosen remedy too frequently or prescribing in too high a potency may result in needless aggravation or accidental proving of the remedy. There is potential danger of an accidental proving taking place when a person continues to take a remedy that was never indicated and exhibits new symptoms, unaware that these have been brought on by the remedy. These symptoms may disappear of their own accord once the person discontinues the remedy, but may require professional homeopathic help to antidote the remedy.

The remedy Thuja, available in health food shops as a remedy for warts, is in fact a very deep-acting remedy used by homeopaths to target the Sycosis miasm of excess. It is therefore frequently indicated for all types of excessive growth or proliferation of tissue, e.g. warts, moles, cysts, hyperplasia and tumours. Because of its sphere of action, there is a possible increased risk of miscarriage, with the body rejecting the fetus, treating it as it would any other growth while under the influence of this remedy. It is therefore best avoided altogether during the first trimester and should only be used with extreme caution by the woman's own homeopath, who will be familiar with all aspects of her case.

The other potential danger occurs when a client, having firmly put their faith in homeopathy, refuses to accept that the time has come for emergency conventional treatment or surgery and that there are some limitations as to what can be treated, e.g. in cases requiring immediate hospitalization or where surgery has become essential. Examples include acute appendicitis, cases of obstruction, removal of mechanical lesions or stones, the repair of congenital defects or orthopaedics. Midwifery exam-

ples include placental abruption and footling breech (it is usually possible to turn most other types of breech in 2–3 weeks using homeopathy).

This does not mean that homeopathy cannot be used in emergency situations, but it is always safer to call out the doctor or ambulance and treat homeopathically on the way to the hospital if necessary. The homeopathy will again become useful in aiding recovery.

How homeopaths prescribe

Homeopathy is practised in many different ways.[8] Some homeopaths have moved away from the principles as laid down by Hahnemann and may, for example, no longer use the 'holistic' approach or else prescribe mixtures of remedies (polypharmacy). Classical homeopathy follows Hahnemann's principles closely and this book is based on the classical approach.

In seeking to cure, homeopaths are guided by the fixed principles, their perception of the vital force, susceptibility and the similar and stronger stimulus. They seek to treat the 'whole person' because symptoms, diseases or pains do not exist in isolation, but reflect how the whole person is coping with stress on all levels of being, i.e. physical, mental, emotional, spiritual or sociological. The homeopath therefore looks beyond the presenting complaint and disease label to find the 'totality of symptoms' that the person presents on all these levels. From the outset of the homeopathic interview, the practitioner gathers vital clues to the required remedy by observation and questioning.

The way in which case taking and analysis are carried out will differ depending on whether the presenting problem is chronic (showing no tendency to ultimate recovery if untreated) or acute (self-limiting), as well as on the person themselves.

A chronic situation will require constitutional treatment, where the homeopath's purpose is to find the 'underlying' person with the disease as opposed to finding out which named disease the person is suffering from or how that alone is being experienced. The constitutional remedy is the one which most closely matches the person on all levels of being and may change during the course of treatment in some cases or remain constant throughout life in others. The gathering of all necessary information involves an in-depth interview exploring not only how the person experiences their complaint (in very great detail) but their personal history, current medication (both prescribed and over the counter), family history, food preferences, thirst, physical general symptoms, menstrual history, perspiration, other discharges, e.g. diarrhoea, etc., sleep and dreams and mental/emotional symptoms. Questions relating to sexual function may be

---

*Alternative toothpastes include Tom's, Hollytrees, Weleda and Kingfisher in a variety of flavours including fennel, salt, bicarbonate of soda, etc.

unnecessary in some cases, but required in others. The order in which the questions are asked depends very much on the person and the degree of rapport with their practitioner, as well as on the nature of the presenting complaint. The outcome of the interview governs the process of remedy selection as well as management of the case, which must both be tailored to each individual client. The remedy will often be prescribed in a medium (e.g. 30C) or high potency (e.g. 1M) and may need to be repeated at infrequent intervals. (Most homeopaths will arrange a first follow-up appointment for 4–6 weeks after giving a remedy to check progress.)

In an acute situation the severity of the condition dictates the time available and hence the form of the case-taking procedure. Again there will be the need to individualize but questioning will concentrate more on the presenting condition – its mode of onset, causation, exact location, the person's sensitivity to factors such as light and noise, etc., modalities (what makes the situation better or worse), fever, perspiration, thirst and appetite, bowel and urinary function, sleep, dreams and state of mind. If the person is undergoing homeopathic constitutional treatment at the time, the homeopath will have to decide whether the acute situation is related to the chronic and treat accordingly, taking into account relationships of remedies, etc. In an acute situation a remedy is most often prescribed in low (e.g. 3X, 6C) to medium potency (e.g. 30C) and repeated more often because the remedy stimulus is 'used up' in direct proportion to the severity of the situation, e.g. during labour, an acute situation, a dose of 30C may need to be repeated every 5–30 minutes. The remedy picture may also change rapidly, calling for a frequent change in remedy.

THE HIERARCHY OF SYMPTOMS

Having taken the case, the homeopath sorts through the symptoms to see which best sum up the person as a whole – in other words, those symptoms which characterize the individual, not symptoms common to the disease label. A useful method of doing this is to apply a symptom hierarchy.[20,21]

The most important symptoms are the subjective – those where the patient says 'I think', 'I feel', 'I have', 'I am', 'I do'. The symptoms of least value are those common to the presenting disease, which are only taken into account if they manifest themselves in a striking manner or distinguish themselves by some other peculiarity. Strange, rare and peculiar (SRP) symptoms are of highest rank[22] and these include:

- negative symptoms – something expected that is absent, e.g. aversion to food when hungry;
- peculiar symptoms, e.g. a woman who chatters continously throughout labour, even during contractions;
- peculiar modalities, e.g. burning pains made better from heat;
- peculiar location, e.g. eczema only around the hairline;
- peculiar sensations, e.g. headache like a band around the head;
- extensions of pain, e.g. toothache extending to the eye;
- peculiar start or end to a symptom; e.g. abruptly;
- 'opposite' symptoms, e.g. one cheek red, the other pale;
- concomitant symptoms, e.g. headache accompanied by copious urination;
- 'periodic' symptoms, e.g. headache every Tuesday;
- 'replacement' symptoms, e.g. nosebleeds instead of menses;
- 'alternating' symptoms, e.g. cough alternating with sciatica.

Mental/emotional symptoms affecting the will, understanding and intellect are also of very great value. Symptoms such as impulses to throw things or suicidal tendencies relate to the will. Delusions, fixed ideas, confusion, mistakes in writing and speaking relate to the understanding and intellect. Grief, sadness, excessive cheerfulness, anger, irritability and fears relate to the emotions.

General symptoms are of vital importance not merely because they relate to the person as a whole. They can also be used to distinguish between remedies which may be near-identical in their particular symptoms, yet be opposite in their general symptoms, e.g. Secale and Arsenicum. They include the subjective symptoms mentioned above, as well as the dreams, desires, aversions, special senses and menstruation – those symptoms that relate to the whole being and not simply to part of it. Therefore, if a person describing 'parts' repeats a common theme, say burning pain in the head, the stomach, the feet and the skin, this too is considered general. If the person described burning in the stomach only, this would remain a particular 'my' symptom, of lesser importance. Causes are also of importance, e.g. never well since glandular fever or walking in a cold wind.

The above hierarchy (from most to least important) can be summarized as follows:

- strange, rare and peculiar (SRP) symptoms;
- the will;
- mental and emotional symptoms;
- general symptoms – including sleep, menses, likes, dislikes, time, temperature, weather, position, motion, stimuli, eating, drinking, clothing and bathing;
- causes;

- particular symptoms – especially anything strange or rare. Also modalities of the particulars.

Next, these symptoms are graded and located in the Repertory and cross-referenced so that remedies that do not apply to each symptom can be eliminated. Those remedies that survive this elimination process are then researched in the Materia Medica to find which one's totality best corresponds to that of the person. Having found a match, the person's 'vitality' is assessed in order to find the appropriate potency. The prescription has now been individualized to fit the whole person.

This process may prove lengthy but is worthwhile as, once selected, the correct prescription will bring speedy relief. This is particularly true in an acute situation, e.g. during labour the correct remedy can be expected to act within 1 minute. When treating a chronic disease improvement will be slower, as both the disease process and remedy action occur on a deeper level.

REFERENCES

1. Kunzli J 1982 Organon of medicine, Samuel Hahnemann: a new translation. Gollancz, London, paragraphs 9–12
2. Kunzli J 1982 Organon of medicine, Samuel Hahnemann: a new translation. Gollancz, London, paragraphs 31, 33, 73
3. Kunzli J 1982 Organon of medicine, Samuel Hahnemann: a new translation. Gollancz, London, paragraphs 6, 7
4. Kunzli J 1982 Organon of medicine, Samuel Hahnemann: a new translation. Gollancz, London, paragraphs 77–82
5. Hahnemann S 1989 The chronic diseases, their particular nature and their homoeopathic cure, trans. Tafel L H. Jain, New Delhi
6. Kunzli J 1982 Organon of medicine, Samuel Hahnemann: a new translation. Gollancz, London, paragraphs 46–51
7. Kunzli J 1982 Organon of medicine, Samuel Hahnemann: a new translation. Gollancz, London, footnote to paragraph 56
8. Watson I 1991 A guide to the methodologies of homoeopathy. Cutting Edge Publications, Kendal
9. Kunzli J 1982 Organon of medicine, Samuel Hahnemann: a new translation. Gollancz, London, paragraphs 105–142
10. Kunzli J 1982 Organon of medicine, Samuel Hahnemann: a new translation. Gollancz, London, paragraph 143
11. Sherr J 1993 The homoeopathic proving of chocolate. Dynamis School of Advanced Homoeopathic Studies, Malvern
12. Houghton J, Halahan E 1994 The homoeopathic proving of Lac caninum. Private publication, available through the Homeopathic Supply Company
13. Murphy R 1993 Homeopathic medical repertory – a modern repertory. Hahnemann Academy of North America, Pagosa Springs, Colorado
14. Schroyens F 1993 Synthesis – repertorium homoeopathicum syntheticum. Homoeopathic Book Publishers, London
15. Kunzli J 1982 Organon of medicine, Samuel Hahnemann: a new translation. Gollancz, London, paragraph 269
16. Kunzli J 1982 Organon of medicine, Samuel Hahnemann: a new translation. Gollancz, London, paragraph 273
17. Kunzli J 1982 Organon of medicine, Samuel Hahnemann: a new translation. Gollancz, London, paragraph 275
18. Kunzli J 1982 Organon of medicine, Samuel Hahnemann: a new translation. Gollancz, London, footnote to paragraph 260
19. Kunzli J 1982 Organon of medicine, Samuel Hahnemann: a new translation. Gollancz, London, paragraph 276
20. Kunzli J 1982 Organon of medicine, Samuel Hahnemann: a new translation. Gollancz, London, paragraphs 83–90
21. Kent J T 1987 Lectures on homeopathic philosophy. Thorsons, Wellingborough, Lectures XXXII and XXXIII
22. Kunzli J 1982 Organon of medicine, Samuel Hahnemann: a new translation. Gollancz, London, paragraphs 153–156

FURTHER READING

Blackie M 1986 Classical homoeopathy. Beaconsfield, Beaconsfield, Bucks

Castro M 1990 The complete homoeopathy handbook – a guide to everyday health care. Macmillan, London

Castro M 1992 Homoeopathy for mother and baby – pregnancy, birth and the post-natal year. Macmillan, London

Crockett P 1995 The unfolded organon: a precis of Hahnemann's sixth edition. Islington Centre of Homoeopathy, London

Kent J T 1986 Repertory of the homoeopathic materia medica and a word index, 6th edn. Homoeopathic Book Service, London

Kent J T 1987 Lectures on homoeopathic philosophy. Thorsons, Wellingborough

Koehler G 1986 The handbook of homoeopathy – its principles and practice. Thorsons, Wellingborough

Murphy R 1993 Homoeopathic medical repertory – a modern repertory. Hahnemann Academy of North America, Pagosa Springs, Colorado

Roberts H A 1936 The principles and art of cure by homoeopathy – a modern textbook. Indian Books and Periodicals Syndicate, New Delhi

Schroyens F 1993 Synthesis – repertorium homoeopathicum syntheticum. Homoeopathic Book Publishers, London

Ullman D 1989 Homoeopathy – medicine for the 21st century. Thorsons, Wellingborough

Vithoulkas G 1985 Homoeopathy – medicine of the new man. Thorsons, Wellingborough

Vithoulkas G 1986 The science of homoeopathy. Thorsons, Wellingborough

Watson I 1991 A guide to the methodologies of homoeopathy. Cutting Edge Publications, Kendal

Wright-Hubbard E 1990 A brief study course in homoeopathy. In: Homoeopathy as art and science. Beaconsfield, Beaconsfield, Bucks

Using this book 1.5

The aim of homeopathy is to match an overall picture of an individual to a remedy picture, the 'picture' being a characteristic collection of symptoms.

One of the best ways of gaining useful information about the mother, and the only possible way to do so for the infant, is to remain observant at all times, noting what is seen, felt, heard and smelt. First impressions should not be dismissed, bearing in mind that anything unusual is of greatest importance. Open-ended questions (which cannot simply be answered by 'yes' or 'no') are the most effective in gathering further information.

Particular attention should be paid to the following.

- The woman's emotional state – is she irritable, anxious, weepy, etc? Does she seek comfort and attention or want to be left alone?
- Is she sensitive to movement, touch, pressure, noise, heat or cold? Do these things make her feel better or worse?
- Is there a time of day or night when she feels better or worse?
- Is she hot or cold to the touch and in herself?
- Does she ask for hot or cold drinks or none at all?
- What sort of food and drink does she like or dislike?
- How quickly have the symptoms developed?
- Was there a causative factor such as a shock or exposure to cold or damp?
- On which side of the body did the symptoms first appear and where are they occurring now?
- What does the pain feel like – stinging, burning, cutting, dragging?
- Do any of the symptoms occur in groups, such as nausea when smelling cooking or headache improved after micturition?

This book aims to speed up the process of homeopathic remedy selection by providing tabulated remedy comparisons for various conditions related to pregnancy, labour and the postnatal period. Each remedy described in detail occupies a vertical column of the table; the symptoms for comparison read horizontally and relate to the particular condition. Most tables include descriptions of mental/emotional and general symptoms, as these rank highly in the symptom hierarchy and are frequently of importance. The 'Other Remedies' section included in most tables lists remedies whose characteristics and suggested uses have been briefly outlined in Appendix 1.

The most useful starting point within a table depends on the presenting problem and the points of greatest need within each individual case. During labour, for example, remedies are best selected on the emotional state and not the type of pain, unless

21

this is very marked. In other situations such as haemorrhage, the characteristics of the blood would be the best starting point.

Once a likely remedy has been selected from the table, the choice should be confirmed using the Materia Medica (remedy pictures) section of the book. Each remedy entry in the Materia Medica is set out as follows:

- Popular remedy name:
  - abbreviation as found in homeopathic literature (in brackets)
  - full remedy name
  - other names
- Prime indications – list of the symptoms which together form the 'core' or 'nucleus' of the remedy
- Additional characteristics:
  - *general* – factors relating to the person as a whole
  - *emotional* – traits which may be seen in a person requiring the remedy
  - *caused by* (listed only if marked) – factors to which a person requiring this remedy is most susceptible and which often contribute to the appearance of a complaint
  - *sensations* (listed only if marked) – most frequently experienced and described by the person
  - *pains* (listed only if marked) – adjectives frequently used to describe the pain experienced
- Worse – factors which aggravate
- Better – factors which ameliorate
- Note – additional information, usually relating to the relationship with other remedies
- Suggested uses – listed in alphabetical order, giving source references. A cross-reference list of alternative remedies from the tables, described in the Materia Medica section and Appendix 1, is also given in brackets.

  This list is not exhaustive and absence of a 'suggested use' does not contraindicate the choice of remedy. In any given situation, the remedy with the closest matching overall remedy picture is most likely to be effective.

For example, the remedy Calendula is presented as follows:

Calendula (Calen) *Calendula officinalis*. Other names: Marigold

---

Prime indications:
- **Torn or ragged wounds**
- **Lacerated or suppurating wounds**
- **Injuries where the skin is broken**
- **Inflammation and redness with a great deal of discomfort**
- **Pain is out of proportion to the injury**

Additional characteristics:
General
- Sensitive to cold air, particularly in cloudy weather

Sensations
- As if beaten

Pains
- Rheumatic drawing pains, only during motion

Worse
- Evening
- Damp weather

Better
- Warmth
- Rest

Notes May be alternated with any other remedy that is needed

Suggested uses:
- Episiotomy or tear[3,12] (Acet-ac; Caust; Staph). Calendula tincture can be applied externally by adding a few drops of tincture to a glass of water to speed the healing process. It may sting for a short while! ('Hypercal', a blend of Hypericum and Calendula mother tinctures, is available for the same purpose.)
- After forceps delivery[3] (Arn; Caust; Cham; Hyp; Staph). In this case it is better given internally in potentized form
- Infection of the umbilical cord in an infant who is otherwise healthy[4] (Sil). Best used in aqueous solution and dressed with Calendula ointment afterwards

NB: References in the tables and Materia Medica appear on pp. 132.

If there are no likely remedies described in the main body of the table, then fuller descriptions of remedies listed in the 'Other Remedies' section of the table can be found in Appendix 1 (see also Fig. 1.5.1).

As an example, imagine a mother with the following postpartum problems following a protracted natural labour, during which she sustained a perineal tear (repaired with three stitches). She also had postpartum haemorrhage and now presents with the following:

- exhaustion and weakness;
- sore, cracked nipples, with inadequate lactation;
- subinvolution with offensive lochia;
- sleeplessness, linked to depression, shown by a loss of interest in the welfare of the infant and herself.

She is also:

- complaining that she cannot get warm, yet perspires easily on exertion;

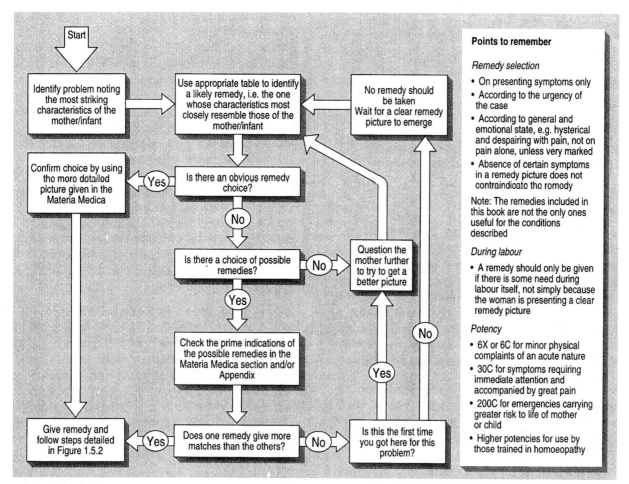

Fig. 1.5.1   Selecting a remedy.

- complaining that she is continually being disturbed by the noise of the baby;
- worse from consolation and sympathy.

The most pressing problem here is the depression, which by its nature is linked to the sleeplessness and exhaustion. In the Depression table, reading across the rows labelled Emotionally and Generally, it can be seen that further details will be required to clarify the emotional state but that from what is known so far, the choice can already be narrowed down to China (exhausted), Cimicifuga (possible as 'unable to sleep after breast-feeding'), Natrum muriaticum (chilly), Sepia (chilly). Checking the rows 'Worse From' and 'Better From' next narrows the choice still further, as Cimicifuga is ruled out.

Now is a good time to clarify the emotional state by asking the mother and/or her partner some more searching questions. Questioning reveals that:

- the woman hides herself away in order to cry;
- she lies on the bed, mulling over the more unpleasant aspects of the labour.

Checking in the Emotional row of the table again, it can be seen that both the descriptions for Natrum muriaticum and Sepia could still be appropriate to this case. Further questioning reveals nothing more of great value, making it necessary to look at more detailed descriptions of both remedies in the Materia Medica section of the book, to see which gives a closer overall match.

The following symptoms match the case under:

Natrum muriaticum

Prime indications:
- **Constant dwelling on past unpleasant occurrences**
- **Depression made worse from consolation**

Additional characteristics:

General chilly; states of weakness accompanied by mental and nervous sensitivity and deep sadness; weakness

Emotional weeping; wants to be alone

Worse consolation

Sepia

Prime indications:
- **Weeping, averse to company**
- **Indifference**
- **Chilly**

Additional characteristics:

General exhausted and run down; perspires easily; extremely sensitive to the cold; weakness

Caused by loss of vital fluids

Worse consolation

So far, it remains unclear which of these two remedies to recommend, but the Suggested Uses show that Natrum muriaticum matches under Postnatal depression only, whereas Sepia matches under Postnatal depression, Sore, cracked nipples and Subinvolution, thus covering more aspects of the case. A glance at the Subinvolution table further confirms that offensive lochia is also covered by this remedy, therefore making Sepia the most probable remedy, going by what is known of the case.

Response to the remedy

- If there is an *improvement* after the first dose, the remedy should be repeated only when the same symptoms return.
- If there is *no change* in the woman (as noticed by either the midwife or the woman herself) after the first dose and the remedy choice is believed to be correct, the remedy should be repeated. If this is *followed by improvement*, the remedy should be repeated only when the same symptoms return.
- If there is *still no improvement*, the case should be reassessed – the wrong remedy may have been selected or the remedy picture may have changed. The same remedy should only be repeated at this stage if the remedy choice is still believed to be correct. If this is *followed by improvement*, the remedy should be repeated only when the same symptoms return.
- If there is *still no improvement*, the remedy chosen is most probably incorrect and should be discontinued to avoid accidental proving.

At this point more information will be required and if possible, the advice of the woman's homeopath should be sought to ascertain whether to change the remedy, change the potency, try the woman's constitutional remedy (if known) (see How Homoeopaths Prescribe section, p. 18), assess the possibility of remedy contamination or antidoting or await further developments. If in doubt, it is better not to let the woman take any more remedy and to continue with conventional or other chosen alternative

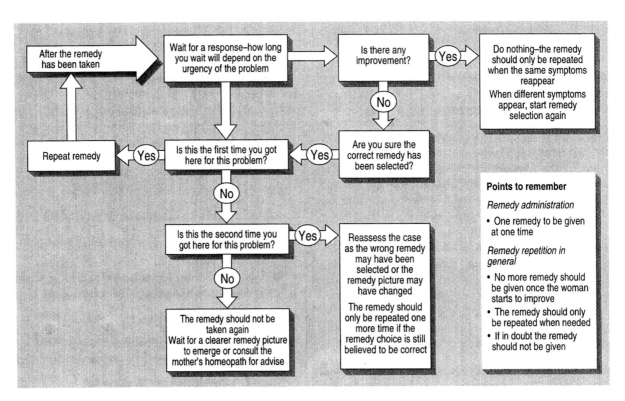

Fig. 1.5.2 Remedy administration.

treatment. The homeopathy may be tried again later during the labour when a clearer or different remedy picture becomes apparent. Alternatively, it may be better to set the homeopathy aside until the recovery period (see also Fig. 1.5.2).

Limitations of this book

Although homeopathy can help in life-threatening situations and in the treatment of serious disease, these situations should only be treated by fully trained and experienced homeopaths. Women with pre-existing conditions such as diabetes, epilepsy, thyrotoxicosis, cardiac disease or other major illnesses, for example cancer, should not be prescribed homeopathic remedies by their midwife. Homeopathy should only be used by their homeopath in conjunction with their consultant obstetrician and physician.

Part 2

Pregnancy

Table 2.1 Abdominal pain

Remedy	Arnica	Arsenicum	Bellis perennis	Bryonia	Cimicifuga
Cause	Active fetus The fetus seems to lie crosswise which causes constant pain	Fetal movements	Uterine ligament tension	Uterine ligament tension	Uterine ligament tension
Pain	Sore Bruised	Burning	Sudden Uterus feels sore	Dull Burning in the fundus uteri	Sharp, shooting Changes location Bruised
Worse from	After eating	After midnight	Towards end of pregnancy	Towards end of pregnancy Evening Movement	Towards end of pregnancy Cold
Better from	Resting	Getting up and moving about	Continued motion	Fresh air	Gentle, continued motion
With	Nausea also caused by motions of the fetus Insomnia caused by the pain	Violent vomiting	Groin pains Stiffness in the lower limbs	Great stiffness in the lower abdomen	
Emotionally/ Generally	Denies feeling unwell Does not want anyone near	Anxious and restless Prefers attentive company	No marked symptoms	Very irritable and touchy Does not want to be interfered with in any way	Very distressed by the pains Depression may alternate with physical symptoms Chilly

Table 2.1 Abdominal pain (Cont'd)

Remedy	Nux vomica	Pulsatilla	Sepia	Staphysagria
Cause	Fetal movements	Fetal movements Malposition of fetus	Fetal movements	Sudden fetal movement
Pain	Dull	Changeable in nature and location	Stitching Shooting	Sudden
Worse from	Morning In bed Midnight	Evening	Cold	After eating
Better from	Getting up and moving about	In sympathetic company In the fresh air	Vigorous exercise	Rest
With	Morning sickness			Shock or anger
Emotionally/ Generally	Nervy Highly sensitive to everything Irritable when questioned	Changeable Gentle, mild and yielding	Run down and exhausted Irritable Chilly Very sensitive to the cold	Easily offended Has a sense of violation or humiliation with resentment Suffers pain very acutely Perspires from exertion
OTHER REMEDIES	Acetic acidum; Cuprum			

Table 2.2 Backache

Remedy	Belladonna	Bryonia	Calcarea carb	Cimicifuga	Kali carb	Kali phos
Description	Lumbar Sudden onset	Lumbar Sudden onset	Lumbar	Lumbar	Lumbar Coccyx	Lumbar
Pains	Dragging down Sensation as if the back is breaking	Stitching on moving Bruised feeling in the back when lying on it	Aching As if sprained	Bruised Sore Rheumatic	Bruised; dragging down Sore; stitching Severe, so that she feels she must lie down immediately	Bruised Sore
With		Muscles sensitive to touch	Back feels weak – soon slumps down in chair	Pains may alternate with depression	Stiffness Sensation of weakness in the back	
Worse from	Jarring movement Touch Pressure	Coughing Slightest movement, e.g. stooping or bending forward	Damp Getting up from sitting	Cold	3 am After long sitting Walking	
Better from	Lying down	Lying down Firm pressure			Lying on hard surface Firm pressure	Movement Warmth
Cause	Relaxin		Lifting	Overexertion		
Emotionally	Agitated Excitable Restless	Irritable Resents intrusion	Anxious and sluggish	Bouts of gloominess alternate with excitability	Touchy, angry, irritable and sluggish	Unreliable memory Anxiety
Generally	Thirsty	Desires cold drinks and hot food	Chilly, with cold clammy hands Sweat on single parts and on head at night	Chilly	Chilly Perspires easily	Nervous exhaustion Startles easily

Table 2.2 Backache (Cont'd)

Remedy	Lycopodium	Natrum mur	Nux vomica	Phosphorus	Pulsatilla	Sepia	Silica
Description	Lumbar	Lumbar	Lumbar	Lumbar Sacral Between shoulder blades	Lumbar Small of back	Lumbar, with pain extending to uterus	
Pains	Sore Sensation as if the back is breaking	Aching Bruised Feels broken Sore	Aching Bruised, as if beaten Dragging down Pressing Sore	Feels broken Burning	Aching Dragging down Pressing	Aching Dragging down As if hit by a hammer	Bruised Sore Stitching
With	Stiffness Trapped wind	Weakness	Weakness Stiffness Desire to defaecate	Weakness	Stiffness	Weakness Stiffness	Weakness Stiffness Lameness
Worse from	Beginning to move Passing stool Getting up from sitting	Raising the arms	In bed Movement Morning	Getting up from sitting Pressure	Getting up from sitting Beginning to move	Afternoon Night Bending down Sitting	Breast-feeding Night Pressure Sitting Getting up from sitting
Better from	Movement Passing wind During micturition	Lying on hard surface Pressure		Massage	Gentle exercise Walking slowly	Hard pressure Walking	
Cause	Lifting	Physical exertion involving bending over for long periods of time	Relaxin Overexertion Getting chilled	Overexertion	Relaxin		Falling to back Injury to coccyx Physical exertion
Emotionally	Capable exterior hides lack of self-confidence	Appears cold and prickly due to difficulty expressing emotions	Nervy Highly sensitive Irritable	Gregarious Craves and gives sympathy Reassured easily	Gentle, mild, yielding, clingy Better weeping in company	Run down and exhausted	Shy Irritable when consoled or feeling low
Generally	Poor digestion Craves sweets	Dryness Extreme thirst	Has to sit up in order to turn over in bed	Chilly Sensitive to changes in weather	Chilly Thirstless Desires air	Chilly Extremely sensitive to the cold	Lacks stamina Easily tired and chilled

OTHER REMEDIES   Ferrum; Hypericum; Mercurius; Zincum

Table 2.3 Carpal tunnel syndrome

Remedy	Apis	Arsenicum	Calcarea carbonica	Causticum	Lycopodium	Sepia
Sensations	Tingling and numbness in fingers and hands, extending upwards	Tingling and numbness in fingers, extending into the shoulders	Tingling and numbness in fingers	Tingling and numbness in fingers	Tingling and numbness in fingers	Tingling and numbness in fingers
With	Swelling of wrist or fingers		Swelling of wrist and fingers		With or without swelling of wrist and fingers	Swelling of wrists especially in the evening. Deformed, brittle nails
Worse	Fingertips. 1st finger (numbness) 2nd finger (tingling). Left hand	Fingertips on side lain on	1st finger 2nd finger 3rd finger	Mornings Fingertips First finger Thumb	Mornings on waking Night 1st finger 2nd finger 3rd finger 4th finger	Evening Night Fingertips
Better from	Motion					Motion Exercise
Emotionally	Irritable and restless. Fear of being alone. Tearful and complaining. Jealous	Anxious and restless. Fear of being alone. Wants to be looked after. Very demanding	Anxious and sluggish. Has difficulty concentrating	Very sensitive and anxious, reacting against injustice – Pessimistic – despairs of getting well	Restless. Full of fear and anxiety beneath an exterior of capability	Weighed down by responsibility and no longer has the resources to cope. Mental and physical 'sag'. Better alone
Generally	Worse for touch, heat and at 3–5 pm	Marked weakness and prostration. Sensitive to cold. Thirsty for sips	Chilliness with profuse perspiration on single parts, especially the head	Great sensitivity to cold. Dislikes sweet food	Feeble physique	Chilly

Table 2.4 Constipation

Remedy	Causticum	Graphites	Kali carb	Lycopodium	Nux vomica
Stools	Soft, despite constipation	Large Knotty Covered with white shreds of mucus Sour odour	Large Hard	Knotty Hard	Large Hard
Desire for stool	Ineffectual	Ineffectual		Ineffectual	Ineffectual and constant
Abdomen	Stitching pains				
With	Pressure in rectum as if faeces lodged there Profuse micturition at night	Sour urine Profuse micturition at night	Pain before stool Unfinished feeling Profuse micturition at night	Flatulence, passing downwards Unfinished feeling Profuse micturition at night	Unfinished feeling Profuse micturition at night
Worse from	Cold Draughts Evening	Cold Night	Soup Coffee 3 am	Heat of room 4–8 pm	After drinking water
Better from	Passing stool when standing	Warmth After eating	Warm weather During the day	Warm drinks	
Generally/ Emotionally	Chilly Pessimistic Despairing of getting well Cries easily	Chilly Apprehensive Tearful	Touchy, anxious, irritable and sluggish all at the same time Highly strung	Anxious and lacking in self-confidence, beneath a capable exterior Cowardly	Nervy, highly sensitive and irritable Impulsive and quarrelsome Irritable when questioned

Table 2.4 Constipation *(Cont'd)*

Remedy	Opium	Phosphorus	Pulsatilla	Sepia
Stools	Small black balls Hard Receding	Slender, long, narrow, dry and tough like a dog's Voided with great difficulty	Changeable Greenish-yellow Watery or slimy	Large Hard
Desire for stool	Absent			Ineffectual
Abdomen				Feels full
With	Unfinished feeling Drowsiness	Debility No pain Icy cold hands and feet	Indigestion	Sensation of a weight or ball in the anus, not relieved by defaecating Profuse micturition at night
Worse from	Heat During and after sleep	Getting chilled	Stuffy room Starchy food Rich food Night Becoming overheated	Forenoon Evening When alone
Better from	Cold things	Cold foods Morning	After eating Fresh air	Exercise
Generally/ Emotionally	Dull, confused and apathetic after a period of exhilaration	Gregarious When ill requires sympathy Reassured easily	Gentle, yielding, mild, emotional Easily moved to laughter or tears Clingy, dependent Desires company	Snappy, indifferent Women who are worn out by too much to do and not enough resources to see them through it
OTHER REMEDIES	Collinsonia; Cuprum; Ignatia; Magnesia muriatica; Magnesia phosphorica; Sabina			

Table 2.5 Cramping in legs and arms

Remedy	Calcarea carb	Chamomilla	Nux vomica	Sepia
Location	Calf Soles of feet Toes Joints Upper limbs Forearm Hand Knee Leg	Toes Leg Calf	Toes Hands Legs Upper limbs Calf Soles of feet when trying to rise Pains radiate over the entire body	Toes Calf Leg Hip Forearm Thigh Soles of feet
Worse from	After walking Pulling on tights On motion When lifting Morning Night In bed Stretching leg in bed	Stretching herself in bed Evening	Drawing up the limbs Daytime Night Midnight Flexing the leg During labour In bed During chill	While walking In bed at night Latter months of pregnancy
Better from	Heat Lying down	Uncovering	Warmth	
Emotionally	Anxious and possibly sluggish, finding it difficult to concentrate when ill	Angry and excitable, tolerating nothing and nobody	Nervy, highly sensitive and irritable Impulsive and quarrelsome Irritable when questioned	Snappy, indifferent and worn out by too much to do and not enough resources to do it
Generally	Chilly, with cold, clammy hands Sour perspiration on head	Unbearable pain may be accompanied by perspiration	Very chilly Upset by slightest draught After overindulgence	Appetite lost during pregnancy
OTHER REMEDIES	Cuprum; Ferrum; Magnesia phosphorica; Zincum			

Table 2.6 Diarrhoea

Remedy	Arsenicum	China	Phosphorus	Pulsatilla
Stools	Watery Very offensive Burning pain after passing stool	With undigested food	Blood-streaked Frequent Watery	Changeable Greenish-yellow Watery or slimy
With	Exhaustion, nausea Great thirst, drinks in sips Icy cold hands and feet	No pain Indigestion or slow digestion	Debility No pain Icy hands and feet	
Worse from	Cold After drinking After eating fruit or cold food After midnight	After eating Afternoon Alternate days Night	Getting chilled	Night Starchy food Rich food Stuffy room Becoming overheated
Better from	Heat		Cold foods Morning	After eating Fresh air
Generally/ Emotionally	Anxious and very restless and demanding Very fearful, especially when alone	Emotionally weary and physically tired Eventually becomes apathetic or depressed	Gregarious When ill requires sympathy Reassured easily	Gentle, yielding, mild and emotional Easily moved to laughter and tears Clingy, dependent Desires company
OTHER REMEDIES	Mercurius			

Table 2.7 Dizziness and fainting

Remedy	Arsenicum	Belladonna	Cimicifuga	Gelsemium	Kali carb
Problem	Dizziness	Dizziness Faintness	Dizziness	Dizziness, with sensation spreading from the occiput	Faintness, has to lie down
With	Nausea Tendency to fall to the right-hand side Inability to walk with the eyes closed	Dizzy sensation spreading from the occiput Headache Anxiety Tendency to fall backwards On lying down, feels that the bed is bouncing up and down	Nausea Vomiting	Dizzy sensation spreading from the occiput Nausea Arms and legs feel as if they are weighted down with lead Diplopia Tendency to fall	Nausea Tendency to fall backwards
Causes	Postural hypotension	Postural hypotension	Postural hypotension	Tiredness	Anaemia
Worse from	Getting up from lying down Closing the eyes Exercising Open air Evening	Getting up from bending down Stooping After eating Night	Getting up from lying down Stooping	Physical exertion Descending the stairs After eating Prolonged standing	Getting up from sitting Turning around rapidly After eating Prolonged standing Evening
Better from		Lying down Open air	Eating Open air	Temporarily after micturition Closing the eyes	
Emotionally/Generally	Anxious and restless Very demanding – wants to be looked after	Agitated Excitable Restless	Sighing and deep sadness 'as if enveloped in a dark cloud' Much sighing Chilly	Apathy Dullness Listlessness	Touchy Angry Irritable Sluggish
	Marked weakness and prostration Sensitive to the cold	Very thirsty		Trembling Exhaustion Seems intoxicated when trying to move	Chilly Perspires easily

Table 2.7 Dizziness and fainting (Cont'd)

Remedy	Natrum mur	Nux vomica	Pulsatilla	Sepia
Problem	Dizziness	Dizziness Faintness, especially from odours and after eating	Dizziness, causing her to lie down Faintness, especially in a warm room	Dizziness Faintness, with sensation of heat during faintness, followed by coldness afterwards
With	Nausea Constipation Tendency to fall forwards	Nausea Constipation Headache Anxiety Tendency to fall	Nausea Tendency to fall forwards or to the left-hand side	Nausea Tendency to fall
Causes	Postural hypotension Anaemia	Postural hypotension	Postural hypotension Anaemia	Postural hypotension Tiredness
Worse from	Getting up from lying down Stooping Tobacco smoke Walking Mental exertion Evening	Getting up from lying down or sitting In bed Stooping Tobacco smoke Walking Mental exertion Loss of sleep	Getting up from bending down or sitting Stooping Stuffy room Walking Prolonged standing	Getting up from lying or sitting down In bed Stooping Exercising the arms Stuffy room Closing the eyes Stooping Evening Blowing the nose
Better from	Lying down Resting Cold applications	Standing	Fresh air	Cold air Before a thunderstorm
Emotionally/ Generally	Has difficulty expressing emotions Worse from consolation Dryness Extreme thirst	Nervy Highly sensitive Irritable Very chilly	Gentle Mild Emotionally changeable Chilly Thirstless Wants fresh air	Exhausted by responsibilities Worse from sympathy Chilly Extremely sensitive to the cold
OTHER REMEDIES	Ignatia; Laurocerasus			

Table 2.8 Frequency of micturition

Remedy	Arsenicum	Belladonna	Causticum	Natrum mur	Pulsatilla	Sepia
Urging	Bladder as if paralysed	Sensation of motion in the bladder, as of a worm	Loss of sensibility on micturition		Painful Constant, with pressure and tension in the abdomen	Constant with dragging-down pain in pelvis
Micturition	Burning, involuntary Feeling of weakness in abdomen after micturition	Profuse Involuntary	Involuntary during first sleep at night	Involuntary	Involuntary at night, while coughing or passing flatus	Slow getting started Involuntary during first sleep or while coughing
Urine	Proteinuria Burning Scanty	Dark Turbid Haematuria where no pathological condition can be found Proteinuria		Proteinuria		Dark Cloudy Scanty With sediment Proteinuria
Pain			Just after micturition		Burning during and after micturition Spasmodic pain in bladder after micturition	Pressing
Worse from	Cold Cold drinks and food	Touch Lying down	Getting chilled Laughing, sneezing, coughing or walking	Laughing, sneezing or walking	Laughing, sneezing or walking Lying down	Laughing, sneezing or walking
Better from	Heat Warm drinks	Sitting semi-erect	Damp, wet weather			
Generally/ Emotionally	Anxious and restless Great fear with cold sweat Despairs that things will not improve Wants to be cared for Dislikes disorder and confusion	Sudden onset of symptoms Woman has hot, red skin, flushed face, glaring eyes, throbbing carotids, excited mental state and hyperaesthesia of all senses	Intensely sympathetic, suffers the pains of others Pessimistic Fights injustices	Unable to pass urine if other people are present Chilly Introverted – wants to be alone and asks for nothing	Changeable and affectionate Mild, clingy and weepy	Irritable and indifferent to loved ones Feels cold even in a warm room

Table 2.9 Gestational hypertension

Remedy	Apis	Arsenicum	Belladonna	Calcarea carbonica	Gelsemium	Kali carb

With	Proteinuria
	Oedema – ankles
	      feet
	      hands
	      fingers
		Proteinuria
		Oedema
			Proteinuria
			Oedema
				Oedema – ankles
				      feet
				      hands
				      fingers
					Proteinuria	Proteinuria
						Oedema
						(of the left foot only)

Onset			Sudden		Slow	
Worse from	Heat Touch 3–5 pm	After midnight Cold Damp	Touch 3 pm	Draughts Cold Damp	Sweating Micturition	Overheating Uncovering 2–4 am
Better from	Cold	Heat Warm drinks Lying down	Lying down	Lying down Heat	Physical exertion	Warmth of bed
With	Intolerance to heat	Palpitations	Throbbing carotids			
Emotionally	Irritable Tearful Fidgety Fear of death	Anguish Anxious restlessness Fear of death	Wild look Anxious, angry and confused	Anxious Sluggish Difficulty concentrating	Weary – wants to be left alone Sluggish Anticipatory anxiety	Touchy, angry Irritable Sluggish
Generally	Tired, as if bruised all over	Wants to be warmly wrapped	Very sensitive to noise or jarring movement	Weak and breathless on exertion Perspiration on single parts	Weary, trembles with exhaustion	Weak, weary and often anaemic

Table 2.9 *Gestational hypertension* (Cont'd)

Remedy	Lycopodium	Natrum mur	Opium	Phosphorus	Pulsatilla	Sepia
With	Proteinuria Oedema – ankles feet hands fingers	Proteinuria Oedema – ankles feet hands fingers	Oedema	Proteinuria Oedema	Proteinuria Oedema – ankles feet hands fingers	Proteinuria Oedema
Onset						
Worse from	Tight clothes 4–8 pm	After eating Physical exertion 10 am	Warmth of bed	Cold	Cold Stuffy rooms	Cold Night
Better from	Fresh air Warmth of bed	Lying down After perspiration	Open air	Warmth Massage	Fresh air Bathing Crying	Exercise
With						
Emotionally	Anxious and worried due to lack of self-confidence Capable exterior	Difficulty expressing emotions Moods may alternate	Fear, shock and fright that remain	Anxious, fearful, impressionable and imaginative	Changeable, mild, weepy and clingy	Sad, weepy, irritable, quarrelsome May dread to be alone and be worse for company
Generally	Craves sweets Poor digestion, with much bloating	Dislikes the thought of food during pregnancy Thirsty	Complete absence of pain	Thirst for cold drinks Chilly Empty feeling in abdomen	Changeable symptoms Thirstless	Exhaustion Intolerant of noise or pressure of clothing

OTHER REMEDIES **Oedema:** Acetic acidum; Ferrum; Mercurius; Zincum. **Proteinuria:** Ferrum; Helonias; Mercurius; Sabina. **Hypertension in pregnancy:** Mercurius

NOTES Although homeopathy may be used alongside conventional antihypertensive medication, the woman may respond unusually quickly to the conventional treatment as a result. It is therefore essential to monitor the woman's progress with extra care.
Remedies useful for hypertension in labour include: Aconite; Apis; Arnica; Belladonna; Chamomilla; Cimicifuga; Gelsemium; Ignatia; Mercurius; Natrum muriaticum; Opium; Pulsatilla; Sepia.

Table 2.10 Haemorrhoids

Remedy	Arsenicum	Kali carb	Lycopodium	Natrum mur	Nux vomica	Pulsatilla	Sepia	Staphysagria
Description	Bluish/purple Burning Blind Congested Large	Congested Large Grape-like	Bluish/purple Chronic Large	Large	Burning Blind Congested Large Grape-like	Blind Congested Large	Hard Large Grape-like	Ulcerating
External/ Internal	External Internal	External Internal Protrude during defaecation and/or micturition	External Internal Protrude during defaecation	External	External Internal Protruding	External Internal	External Internal Protrude during defaecation	
Pain	Extreme	Extreme	Extreme	Extreme	Extreme	Extreme	Extreme	Extreme
With	Bleeding Debility	Bleeding Stitching sensation in rectum on coughing	Bleeding profusely Moist, itchy skin eruption surrounding the anus Constipation	Constipation Sheep dung-like stools	Constipation Large, hard stool Backache Tenesmus	Bleeding Itching Continual oozing	Bleeding Constipation Continual oozing Sensation of a ball in the rectum	Constipation Itching
Worse from	Latter months of pregnancy	Latter months of pregnancy Touch After delivery	Latter months of pregnancy Touch	Latter months of pregnancy Motion	Latter months of pregnancy Touch In bed at night	Latter months of pregnancy After delivery	Latter months of pregnancy After delivery	Touch After difficult labour or forceps delivery
Better from	Bathing in warm water		Bathing in warm water		Bathing in cold water			Warmth
Emotionally	Very restless and anxious Fear of being alone Wants to be looked after Difficult and demanding	Touchy, angry, irritable and sluggish Easily startled by noise Desires company, whom she treats badly	Capable front hides a lack of self-confidence	Difficulty expressing emotions, so appears hard and prickly	Nervy, highly sensitive and irritable, especially when questioned Impulsive and quarrelsome	Gentle, mild, yielding and emotional Clingy, desiring company and consolation	Responds badly to sympathy Torpor from being worn out	Offended easily, resentful but suppresses her emotions until they are finally released in a violent outburst
Generally	Very sensitive to cold Desires fresh air Tires suddenly	Chilly Very weak and weary Perspires easily and catches cold easily	Chilly Craves sweets	Chilly Dryness and extreme thirst Dislikes hot weather	Very chilly Upset by slightest draught	Chilly Dislikes stuffy rooms Thirstless	Chilly Extremely sensitive to cold Perspires easily Run-down and exhausted	Hyper-sensitive to pain

OTHER REMEDIES   Collinsonia; Hamamelis; Hypericum; Ignatia; Sabina

Table 2.11 Heartburn

Remedy	Bryonia	Calcarea carb	Carbo veg	Causticum	Natrum mur	Nux vomica	Pulsatilla
Eructations	Bitter Empty Sour Taste of food just eaten	Empty Sour	Bitter Empty Foul Nauseous Rancid	Empty Fatty or greasy Taste of food just eaten	Sweetish Watery Incomplete/ ineffectual/ sour or bitter Taste of food just eaten	Bitter Sour Herb-like Difficult With metallic taste in the mouth	Bitter Sour Empty Taste of food just eaten With slimy or salty taste in the mouth
Abdomen		Bloated Hard	Bloated	Feels full		Bloated	Feels empty
Stomach pains		Pressing	Pressing	Pressing Cramping	Pressing Cramping	Pressing Cramping Sore Bruised Heavy, full and tender	Pressing Gurgles and rumbles during the evening
Worse from	Slightest movement After eating Stuffy room Food which causes flatulence	Tight clothing After eating Fresh air Cold	After eating rich or fatty foods Forenoon	Walking Getting wet Evening Cold Draughts	Starchy food After eating	Tight clothing After eating	After supper After eating rich, fatty food, fruit, meat or bread After drinking milk Night
Better from	Lying still	Lying down Being constipated	Eructations	Cold drinks Heat Warmth of bed	Fasting	Hot drinks	Fresh air Keeping busy
Emotionally/ Generally	Irritable, especially when disturbed Does not wish to be interfered with in any way Lips are dry and cracked	Sluggish, breathless and weak on exertion Anxious Concentration difficult	Mentally and physically sluggish Very weak Made worse from extremes of temperature	Pessimistic, despairing of ever getting well Cries easily Chilly	Has difficulty expressing emotions Appears hard yet is very sensitive Cries alone	Nervy, highly sensitive and irritable, especially when questioned Impulsive and quarrelsome	Gentle, yielding, mild, emotional and easily moved to laughter or tears Desires sympathetic company

OTHER REMEDIES   Acetic acidum; Mercurius; Zincum

Table 2.12 Insomnia

Remedy	Aconite	Belladonna	Bellis perennis	Coffea	Gelsemium
Causes	Anxiety Fright Nervousness Restlessness	Anxiety Overactive mind Twitching limbs Acute hearing – hears distant sounds	Getting cold when heated Accident Injury	Cramping Overactive mind – rush of ideas, making plans Overexcitement Good news Nervousness Acute hearing	Nervous irritation Overactive mind – rush of ideas Violent itching of the head, face, neck and shoulders
Sleep	Restless Starts during Light – hears every sound Anxious	Jerking on falling asleep Deep Wakes screaming	Sleeps well until 3 am, after which she cannot sleep	Inclined to lie down and shut the eyes without being able to sleep Light Wakes at every sound May sleep well until 3 am, after which she dozes	Restless Delirious Half-waking Murmuring
Dreams	Anxious Vivid Confused	Nightmares Quarrels, fire and other dangers Of falling		Vivid Long Confused	Unpleasant Of death Disturbing
Sleeping position	On the back with hand under head or Sitting posture with head inclined forward	Sitting posture with the head inclined backwards			
With	Constant tossing	Sleepiness	Sleepiness		Sleepiness during the day Yawning, Headache Colic
Emotionally	Extremely distressed Anxious Fearful	Lively and entertaining when well, but violent when ill	No marked symptoms	Excessive euphoria yet the slightest pain will induce despair	Dull, sluggish Wants to be left alone
Generally		Oversensitivity of all the nerves		Sensitive to the least noise Note: Also useful for insomnia after delivery	Weary Exhausted

Table 2.12 Insomnia (Cont'd)

Remedy	Kali carb	Nux vomica	Opium	Pulsatilla
Causes	Anxiety Active mind Twitching of limbs Itching Exertion	Cramps during pregnancy Excitement Mental strain Overactive mind – rush of ideas Nervousness Acute hearing – overhears distant sounds	Shock Fright Overactive mind – rush of ideas Acute hearing — overhears very distant sounds	Fright Overexcitement Twitching Itching skin (no eruption present) Overactive mind – fixed ideas and continually repeating thoughts
Sleep	Waking between 2 am and 4 am Restless	Waking at midnight or at around 3 am. She then goes back into deep sleep, after which it is almost impossible to wake her at the required time Groans, talks and weeps during sleep	Catnaps Drowsy at first but sleepless afterwards Light Restless Hears every sound Jerking during sleep	Catnaps Restless Waking before midnight Frequent waking Sleeps late in the mornings Chatters during sleep
Dreams	Frightful nightmares Ghosts Anxious	Amorous Misfortune Business of the day	Amorous Fantastic, pleasant or anxious	Anxious, business of the day Vivid, pleasant or frightful – of misfortune
Sleeping position	Sitting up	On the back with her arms raised over her head	On the back with the limbs drawn up	Lies on the back with knees raised and arms over the head or crossed over the abdomen or Unable to sleep except when seated with the head inclined forward or to one side
With	Sleepiness	Sleepiness during the day and on going to bed, but is woken by anxious thoughts	Sleepiness during the day, but wakeful at night Terrific shocks in the limbs during sleep	Sleepiness during the afternoon and evening Sensation of heat after waking
Emotionally		Nervy Highly sensitive Irritable	Stupor preceded by exhilaration As if in a dream	Changeable Gentle Mild Clingy Weepy
Generally	Note: Particularly useful during the third trimester	Morning is her worst time of day, especially after a disturbed night	Blunted senses Lack of pain	Numbness on waking Thirstless Desires fresh air
OTHER REMEDIES	Conium; Ignatia; Rescue remedy			

Table 2.13 Ligament pain/sciatica

Remedy	Arnica	Bellis perennis	Causticum	Phytolacca	Pulsatilla	Sepia
Sensations	Soreness		Numbness	Numbness		
With	Soreness in symphysis pubis or sacroiliac symphysis	Soreness of uterus – feels squeezed	Limping Unsteady gait			
Pains	Bruised Sore	Sudden	Tearing	Run from hip downward Mostly on outer side of the thighs	Changeable in nature	
Worse	Touch Approach	Left leg	Cold Left leg On coughing	Motion Evenings Right side Night	Motion Evenings Warm room	Right leg Forenoon Night In bed Coughing
Better from			Warmth of bed / warmth	Pressure	Fresh air	Walking
Emotionally	'Nothing wrong' Does not wish to be touched or examined	No marked symptoms	Suffers the pain of others Fights injustice Pessimistic	Worn out Exhausted	Clingy Dependent Emotional Weepy Better for consolation	Indifferent to loved ones Wants to be alone Uncommunicative
Generally	After injury	Tired – wants to lie down	Chilly Dislikes anything sweet	Feels she must move, but motion aggravates	Thirstless Desires fresh air	Chilly Feels better during and after physical exertion

OTHER REMEDIES   Ferrum; Magnesia phosphorica

Table 2.14 Loss of libido

Remedy	Causticum	Graphites	Natrum mur	Sepia
With		Strong aversion to coitus	Aversion to husband	Strong aversion to husband – unable to tolerate even his smell
Enjoyment	Absent	Absent	Absent	Absent
Orgasm			Painful	
Pain	Biting	Biting, burning in vagina Vagina very dry	Burning in vagina Vaginal during intercourse Vagina very dry	Vaginal during intercourse intense enough to prevent coitus Vagina very dry – burning pain
Generally/ Emotionally	Chilly Sympathetic – feels the pains of others Fights injustices Pessimistic	Worse from cold in general, but also worse in a warm room Irresolute and full of doubts Always anticipating difficulties	Mainly warm and made worse by heat and consolation Dwells on past unpleasant events Wishes to be on her own	Chilly, even in a warm room Indifferent to loved ones. No longer able to give love and affection Wishes to be on her own

Table 2.15 Nausea and vomiting

Remedy	Antimonium tartaricum	Arsenicum	Ipecacuanha	Nux vomica	Phosphorus
Nausea	Deathly Anxious Comes in waves	Deathly Retching	Constant – unrelieved by vomiting Deathly Empty eructations	Constant – relieved after vomiting After eating Dry heaves	After food and drink have become warmed in the stomach (about 15 minutes) Sour eructations
Sensations as if			Stomach hanging down	Heavy weight in the stomach after eating	'All gone' sensation in the abdomen not relieved by eating Heat between shoulder blades
Vomiting	Forcible – followed by exhaustion and sleep Violent Frequent – bitter or sour	Without nausea Bile Food Frequent, easy, violent Watery, malodorous	Bile Food Difficult retching	Bile, waterbrash Mucus Inability to vomit Retching Bitter, sour, offensive	Bile Mucus Yellow Bitter Violent
Taste in the mouth		Bitter		Bad in the morning Bitter or sour	Sour
With	Tongue coating thick white with reddened papillae and red edges Cold clammy perspiration over the whole body Weakness	Red tongue Faintness after vomiting Perspiration during vomiting Diarrhoea Burning in the stomach Desire for sour things and coffee	Clean tongue Excessive salivation Pallid face, covered in cold perspiration Shortness of breath Thirstlessness	Brown tongue Heartburn Copious saliva Faintness Craving for stimulants	Craving for ice cold drinks and salt Aversion to tea, coffee, boiled milk or meat Weakness Burning pain
Worse from	After vomiting After eating or drinking Night	After vomiting After drinking Cold drinks Ice cream Smell of food Afternoon	After vomiting Immediately after eating Rich food Ice cream Smell of food or tobacco smoke Bending down Warmth Coughing Movement	Immediately after eating Pressure of clothes Morning in bed Perspiring Smell of tobacco smoke	Hot drinks Putting the hands in warm water Sight of water, which brings on nausea
Better from	Lying on the right-hand side	Heat, warm drinks	Open air, cold drinks	After vomiting	
Emotionally	Fearful of being on her own when vomiting Inclined to sleep	Anxious and restless	Anxious After anger or frustration	'If only I could vomit I'd be better' Violent disposition Irritable and angry Sensitive, especially to odours and noise	Fearful Requires sympathy when ill Easily comforted and reassured Gregarious

Table 2.15 *Nausea and vomiting* (Cont'd)

Remedy	Pulsatilla	Sepia
Nausea	Not relieved by vomiting	Intermittent Gnawing pains
Sensations as if		Dragging down in abdomen Empty feeling
Vomiting	Bitter	Bile Malodorous
Taste in the mouth	Bad in the morning Bitter	Bitter Sour
With	Moist white tongue Desire for sour, refreshing things Aversion to fatty foods and meats, bread and milk	Backache Chloasma Desire to vomit again immediately after vomiting Desire for vinegar, sour things, sweets and wine Aversion to bread, fatty food, milk
Worse from	After eating or drinking Coughing Hot drinks Ice cream Rich or fatty food Fruit Stuffy room Morning	Minimal effort, e.g. getting out of bed Company Not eating Smell or thought of food Morning Before breakfast 3–5 pm
Better from	Fresh air, cold drinks	Temporarily better after eating
Emotionally	Mild, yielding, easily moved to laughter or tears Easily hurt	Snappy and indifferent due to exhaustion
OTHER REMEDIES	Acetic acidum; Aletris farinosa; Gossypium	

Table 2.16 Threatened abortion and vaginal bleeding

Remedy	Aconite	Apis	Arnica	Belladonna	Caulophyllum	Cimicifuga	Ipecacuanha
Gestation	Any time	4–16	Any time	12–16	1–12	12	6
Predisposing factors	Fright Anger	Constipation Ovarian disease Oliguria	Shock or injury, concussion, fatigue	Abuse of stimulants or narcotics	Passive uterine congestion Hysteria Rheumatism Uterine inertia Prostration	Uterine congestion Fright Rheumatism Uterine inertia or atony	Emotional shock
Flow	Active	Profuse Dark	Profuse Continuous Bright red Coagulated or serous mucus	Profuse Hot Bright red and clotted or dark red in sudden gushes	Scanty Passive		Profuse, continuous and steady Bright red blood Coagulating in clots
Process and pains		Stinging pain in ovarian region becoming more and more frequent until uterine contractions are produced. The flow then begins. Labour-like in uterine region Extending to thighs	Sensation as if the fetus is lying crosswise in the abdomen Sore and bruised in uterine region	Shooting back pains come and go suddenly Sensation as if back would break	Irregular contractions Spasmodic bearing down Cramping in the abdomen centred low down in the pelvis Severe and tormenting Back pain	Habitual in women with rheumatic tendencies Followed by subinvolution Cramping pains in the abdomen fly from side to side Double her up In back extend to thighs	Haemorrhage predominates Spasms without consciousness Cutting about the umbilicus from left to right, passing off into the uterus With nausea
Worse from	Night Touch		Jarring movement Touch Motion	Jarring movement Touch	Night		
Better from	Fresh air			Lying down			
Generally/ Emotionally	Anxious restlessness Dizzy Thirsty Hot sweat on covered parts Fear of death or that something bad will happen	Yawning Restless Thirstless Fear of being alone Tearful and whining	Head hot and body cold Insists she is fine and does not wish to be touched or examined	Very sensitive to light, noise or jar Dizzy Anxious, angry and confused, with wild appearance	Weakness and trembling Possible history of spontaneous abortion Fearful Irritable Apprehensive	Cold chills with pricking sensation in mammae	Coldness Dyspnoea Continuous nausea without relief Sulky, wants something, but knows not what

Table 2.16 Threatened abortion and vaginal bleeding (Cont'd)

Remedy	Kali carb	Kali phos	Nux vomica	Opium	Pulsatilla	Secale	Sepia
Gestation	8–12 or 20–36	Any time	12–16	Any time or after 32nd	1–12 or 32–36	12–16 or 20–36	12–16 or 20–36
Predisposing factors	Constipation Anaemia	Anaemia Exhaustion	Abuse of stimulants or narcotics Constipation Uterine congestion	Fright Emotional shock, especially in the third trimester	Injury Fright Grief Getting feet wet	Grande multigravida Fright Anaemia Uterine inertia or atony Passive uterine congestion	From least cause Uterine congestion Lax tissue Leucorrhoea
Flow			Scanty		Changeable Stops and starts, becoming more profuse when reappears Clotted black or bright red	Active Black Brown or bright red Fetid – thin with offensive clots	Dark red
Process and pains	Pain predominates Stitching pains begin in the back, spread to buttocks and extend down the thighs Sensation the as if back would break		Pain predominates Spasmodic in uterine region	Pain predominates	Pain predominates Haemorrhage alternates with the pains	Haemorrhage predominates Labour-like pains alternate with the haemorrhage Holds her fingers spread apart Followed by tearing pains in the limbs	Pain predominates Habitual Fetal movements are feeble Colicky pain in uterine region. Sensation of weight in the anus like a heavy ball
Worse from	Eructations Warmth	Cold draughts	3 am	Getting up Warmth of bed		Heat Motion	
Better from		Warmth			Fresh air Weeping Consolation	Cold bathing	Exercise Warm room
Generally/ Emotionally	Backache when walking Feels must sit or lie down Weak, weary and often anaemic With nausea	Very sensitive to the cold Anxious, timid and easily startled Irritable and tearful – wants to be left alone	With constant ineffectual desire to defaecate or micturate Afraid to be moved Irritable and wants to be left alone	Absence of pain Very sleepy, yet is unable to sleep Restless – the sheets feel too hot for her	Thirstless Wants windows open and plenty of company to offer their sympathy and support Mild, weepy and apologetic	Wishes to remain uncovered Wants fresh air Tingling sensation over entire body, better from rubbing Coldness Anxious stupor	Chilly Perspires profusely Flushes of heat with faintness and momentary attacks of blindness Irritable Exhausted Indifferent to loved ones

OTHER REMEDIES   **Abortion**: Alteris farinosa; Ferrum; Gossypium; Helonias; Trillium pendulum. **Bleeding**: Ignatia; Sabina; Trillium pendulum

Table 2.17 Vaginal discharge

Remedy	Natrum mur	Pulsatilla	Sepia
Discharge	Acrid Burning Like egg white Profuse Thick White Watery Yellow	Acrid Bland Burning Cream-like Milky Profuse Slimy, mucous Thick Watery White Yellow	Acrid Brown Burning Cottage cheese-like Like egg white Lumpy Milky Offensive Profuse Thick Watery White Yellow
With	Itching	Itching	Itching and vaginal and vulval dryness or rawness Discomfort from coitus Sensation of dragging down
Worse from	Physical exertion Mid-morning	Heat Stuffy room	Morning Night Cold air
Better from	Lying down	Fresh air	Exercise
Thirst	Extreme, for large quantities	Thirstless	Desires vinegar
Generally/ Emotionally	Has difficulty expressing emotions She is sensitive, yet appears hard Cries alone	Gentle, yielding and mild. Changeable Emotional and easily moved to laughter or tears Clingy, desires company and consolation	Snappy and indifferent Women worn out by too much to do and lack of resources to do it Weepy, may wish to be alone
OTHER REMEDIES	Borax; Helonias; Mercurius. **Pruritus vulvae remedies:** Aconite; Arsenicum; Belladonna; Borax; Calcarea carbonica; Coffea; Collinsonia; Graphites; Hamamelis; Helonias; Lycopodium; Mercurius; Sepia; Silica		

Table 2.18 Varicose veins – leg and vulva

Remedy	Bellis perennis	Calcarea carbonica	Carbo veg	Lycopodium	Nux vomica	Pulsatilla	Sepia
Location	Vulva	Leg Thigh Labia majora Vulva	Leg Thigh Vulva	Leg Thigh Ankles Vulva	Leg Vulva	Upper limbs Leg Thigh Foot	Legs Thigh Around ankles Vulva
Pains	Throb and ache if squeezed Bruised soreness Inability to walk Uterus feels sore – as if squeezed	Burning Soreness		Painful Possible ulceration		Heaviness Stinging Sensitive Limbs lain on become numb Possible bleeding and ulceration	Heaviness in legs, as if paralysed Stiff and unwieldy
Worse from	Pregnancy Left side Heat	Pregnancy Cold	Pregnancy Exertion Lying down	Pregnancy Extremes of heat and cold	Touch Walking	Pregnancy Getting cold Prolonged standing	Morning After sleep
Better from	Cold bathing	Heat		Fresh air	Lying down	Weeping Movement Pressure Open air Cold applications	
Emotionally		Anxious and possibly sluggish, finding it difficult to concentrate when ill	Anxious in late afternoon, which intensifies when she goes to bed and shut her eyes Sluggish Low vitality	An aura of capability hides a lack of confidence	Nervy, highly sensitive and irritable Impulsive and quarrelsome	Mild, yielding and apologetic	Snappy and indifferent, due to exhaustion from many responsibilities
Generally	A useful remedy after accident or surgery to aid recovery	Chilly, with cold, clammy hands and sweat on head	Feels easily worn out Must have fresh air	Chilly Craves sweets	Very chilly Upset by slightest draught After overindulgence	Thirstless Desires fresh air	Appetite lost during pregnancy

OTHER REMEDIES   Ferrum; Hamamelis; Trillium pendulum; Zincum

NOTE Hamamelis may be useful for varicose veins of the legs when there are no clear indications for another remedy.

Part 3

Labour

Table 3.1 Emotional shock

Remedy	Aconite	Arnica	Opium	Phosphorus	Staphysagria
Process	Mother shaky from shock Baby lies very still with fear in its eyes	Does not want to be touched Denies she is unwell Suffers bad dreams	Dream-like stupor, that she cannot snap out of Recreates the cause of the shock during waking hours	Requires sympathy Despite her fears is easily comforted and reassured	Feelings of having been mentally or physically assaulted Suppressed feelings may turn into anger and resentment
Cause	Anaesthetic Injury Surgery Precipitate delivery	Injury Delivery Surgery	Anaesthetic Injury Surgery	Surgery	Injury Surgery
With	Anxiety Fear Insomnia	Bad dreams	Stupor	Vomiting of bile Fear	Anger Indignation
Worse from	Night Touch	During sleep Touch Lying on injured part	During sleep On getting up Warmth of bed	After eating or drinking Morning Evening	Exertion Fasting Touch Tobacco
Better from	Fresh air	Lying with head low	Uncovering Constant walking	After sleep Massage	Warmth Rest After breakfast

OTHER REMEDIES   Acetic acidum; Hypericum; Ignatia; Rescue remedy

Table 3.2 Failure to progress

Remedy	Aconite	Arnica	Belladonna	Carbo veg	Caulophyllum
Generally	Fear can stop the contractions Fearful, restless, moaning Anxious expression Parts feel contracted With headache Faintness Intolerant of internal examination	Denies her suffering Restless because feels sore and bruised all over, whatever her position Great distress. Faintness Body feels cold, head feels hot Intolerant of internal examination	Vehement, wild, moaning Desires to escape, enraged Face flushed, red, hot, eyes glisten Great distress, headache Cramps in hands and legs Faintness Exhaustion	Anxious or indifferent Great weakness Faintness	Post-dates Fretful and exhausted, shivering Too weak to develop contractions Fever, thirst during contractions Irritability Trembling (internally) Faintness and nausea
Contractions	Very severe In rapid succession Ineffectual due to malposition of fetus CEASING ENTIRELY from local sensitivity Great soreness in back	Distressing Too weak Irregular Spasmodic CEASING Violent Ineffectual From local sensitiveness Occur on motion of fetus	Distressing Too weak Irregular Spasmodic CEASING Severe Ineffectual Sudden From nervousness Drawing pain from the small of the back to thighs Back feels as if it will break	Too weak CEASING ENTIRELY Shifting from the groins down the legs	Drawing Too weak Distressing Spasmodic CEASING FROM EXHAUSTION Too short Irregular Ineffectual Intermittent Sharp, cramping pain in uterine ligaments, bladder or groin flies in all directions, e.g. down the legs
Fear	That she or the baby will die Remains after the labour		Fearless		
Birth canal	Os – tender, dry, undilatable, rigid, contracted spasmodically, sensitive Cervix – undilatable Vulva – dry Vagina – hot, dry, tender, undilating	Uterus – fatigued	Os – thin, rigid, hot, dry, tender, sensitive, contracted spasmodically Cervix – fails to soften, hot and very dry Vagina – hot, dry, and in spasm	Vulva – varicose	Uterus – lack of tone, even at the height of a contraction Os – rigid, spasmodic contractions Cervix – needle-like pains Vagina – profuse secretion of mucus
Hypertension	Hypertension	Hypertension	Hypertension		
Worse from		Being touched	Noise	Warmth	Cold
Better from				Being fanned	Cool fresh air, back pressed hard
NOTE					Should not be given routinely as can result in either protracted labour or precipitate labour, especially in women with a history of quick, easy labours

Table 3.2 Failure to progress *(Cont'd)*

Remedy	Chamomilla	China	Cimicifuga	Cinnamomum	Coffea
Generally	'I cannot bear it any more' Rude, nervous, moaning, restless Oversensitive to noise and pain Thirsty. Frequent micturition Faintness, dizziness, headache, nausea and exhaustion Refuses internal examination	Cannot bear to be touched during a contraction, especially on the hands Faintness Dizziness Exhaustion	Post-dates. Says she will go crazy, her behaviour may cause concern May think she sees rats Hysterical, melancholy Nervous, complaining, restless Chilliness, twitching, trembling Faintness, headache	Hysterical Twitching Faintness	Feels she will go crazy. Irritable, excitable, full of ideas Restless, despairing, weeping Faintness Chilly with hot head Puffed face
Contractions	Very severe – unbearable Distressing Too weak Irregular CEASING Spasmodic Shifting upwards, beginning in the back Tearing in abdomen, shooting down the inner side of the legs	Too weak CEASING ENTIRELY from nervousness Digging Tearing	Severe Distressing Too weak Ineffectual CEASING ENTIRELY Irregular Spasmodic The contractions can come if the woman is chilled and stop when she becomes warmer Tearing, fly around the abdomen With cramps in the hip	Too weak Ineffectual CEASING ENTIRELY	Severe Distressing Irregular Ineffectual CEASING with talkativeness Spasmodic Worse in the small of the back
Fear	Caused by the severity of pain		Of death Of the birth Of going insane		Of death
Birth canal	Os – rigid Cervix – fails to soften Vagina – dark coagulated blood, burning sensation	Uterine inertia	Os – rigid; now dilated, now closed in spasm Cervix – fails to soften Uterine inertia		Cervix – fails to dilate Vulva – rigid
Hypertension	Hypertension				
Worse from	Noise and pain	Noise	Noise and pain		Draughts
Better from	Cool, fresh air Moving about	Cool, fresh air Being fanned			
NOTES	Tosses about, is hot, perspiring and red-faced With loose stools and flatulence		Talks incessantly, even during a contraction	The placenta may descend with the head Severe flooding in primipara after the first few contractions	May be useful where well-indicated Aconite has failed to help

Table 3.2 *Failure to progress* (Cont'd)

Remedy	Gelsemium	Kali carb	Kali phos	Lycopodium	Natrum mur
Generally	Chatters during first stage Headache Dark, uniformly flushed face after every contraction Trembling hysteria Lack of will-power – exhausted, even at start of labour Nausea in early labour	Obstinate Oversenstive Restless Chilly after contraction Anxiety felt in the stomach Flatulence and bloated abdomen Exhaustion Increased thirst With violent headache	Exhausted Mental tiredness Cannot concentrate on her breathing Exhaustion	Anxious, weeping, while walking around the room Restless, eyes half-closed Dictatorial Exhaustion Flatulent Retention of urine	Does not want to go through with the labour Desires privacy Melancholy Thirsty for cold gulps Exhaustion
Contractions	Distressing Too weak Ineffectual Spasmodic CEASE ENTIRELY when examined Backache labour – cramps in abdomen go through to and up the back, then extend to the hips Shift upwards – fetus seems to ascend with every contraction Occur like a wave, ending in a choking feeling. This and her anxiety impede labour	Distressing Too weak Ineffectual Spasmodic Light touch can stop the contractions CEASING Backache labour – sharp, bearing-down pain from back to pelvis. Cutting in lumbar region Linger and pass down to buttocks	Too weak Slow – every 15–30 min Ineffectual Spasmodic	Distressing Too weak CEASING Spasmodic Going upwards or from right to left The woman finds greatest relief by pressing and relaxing her foot alternately against a support so as to agitate her whole body	Too weak CEASING, from interruption or emotions Spasmodic drawing in back descending to thigh Headache at beginning of labour
Fear	Dreads the delivery Being alone Of the future	Imaginations in general Being alone		Anticipatory anxiety	
Birth canal	Uterine inertia; atony Os – rigid, thick, swollen Cervix – soft, flabby or spasmodically contracted into hard unyielding ring	Uterine inertia Cervix – fails to dilate		Os – rigid, spasmodic contractions Vaginal – dry	Cervix fails to soften Vagina dry
Hypertension	Hypertension				Hypertension
Worse from		Light touch			
Better from	Bending forward, movement	Back pressed hard or rubbed fast		Motion	
NOTE	Becomes dull and sleepy after each contraction and her speech thickens Progress improves after micturition				

Table 3.2 Failure to progress (Cont'd)

Remedy	Nux vomica	Opium	Pulsatilla	Secale	Sepia
Generally	Oversensitive, especially to touch Irritable Nervous Ugly behaviour Premature labour Trembling Headache Faintness and exhaustion Must stand or walk about	Apathetic Fearful, face red and bloated Sleepy Twitching Retention of urine and stool Exhaustion Stupor	Apologetic Changeable – laughing, then weeping Face pale Wants sympathy and to be fanned Great distress Thirstless, with dry mouth Faintness and sleepiness Nausea, vomiting and exhaustion	Stupor Parts open and loose without action Trembling when contractions cease Refuses to be covered Faintness	Snappy, irritable and indifferent Resentful if left 'I've had enough' Cold extremities and flushes of heat Faintness and coldness Wants to be covered up more as she feels this will help her endure the pain
Contractions	Severe Distressing Too weak Irregular Ineffectual CEASING ENTIRELY Backache labour – with spasmodic drawing in back, descending to thighs Cramps in hands or legs With ineffectual urge to micturate or defaecate	Too weak Suppressed, from fear Irregular Ineffectual CEASING ENTIRELY, with coma	Distressing Too short Too weak Irregular Ineffectual CEASING Wandering, shift from the sacrum to the region of the stomach, where they result in vomiting Cutting, pressing Occur on motion of fetus Backache labour – spasms in back appear suddenly and subside gradually	Distressing Too short Too weak Irregular Ineffectual CEASING, after which trembling and twitching begin Spasmodic	Severe Too weak Ineffectual CEASING Spasmodic pains shoot upwards from the cervix Felt in the back Sensation of weight in the anus Contractions are accompanied by shuddering
Fear	Fright may cause premature labour	Dread of suffocation			
Birth canal	Os – rigid, with spasmodic contractions during first stage Cervix – fails to soften, constrictive pain		Intense uterine inertia Cervix – fails to dilate	Uterine inertia; atony Os – rigid, spasmodic contractions Cervix – fails to soften There is no expulsive effort, even though everything seems loose and wide open	Cervix – hard Os – rigid, spasmodic contractions Great tenderness of anterior lip Vagina dry, in spasm
Hypertension		Hypertension	Hypertension		Hypertension
Worse from	Noise, draught of fresh air	While perspiring; bed feels too hard		Being covered	
Better from	Warm room, back pressed hard	Constant walking, fresh air	Company, fresh air, walking about	Cool fresh air, being uncovered	Being covered, warmth

Table 3.2 Failure to progress (Cont'd)

Remedy	Nux vomica	Opium	Pulsatilla	Secale	Sepia
NOTE			If no other remedy is clearly indicated, Pulsatilla may be used to correct malpresentations before the presenting part is engaged or before the membranes are ruptured		

OTHER REMEDIES **Failure to progress:** Borax; Cuprum; Ignatia; Magnesia muriatica. **Nausea during labour:** Ipecac. **Hypertension during labour:** Apis; Ignatia; Mercurius

NOTE The woman's constitutional remedy (if known) may succeed in making the labour progress.

Table 3.3 Fear

Remedy	Aconite	Arsenicum	Calcarea carbonica	Cimicifuga
Occurrence	Pregnancy/labour	Night/labour	Evening	During pregnancy
Fears	Of death during pregnancy On walking across a busy street In a crowd	Fear of vomiting That a friend has met with an accident Death; robbers Being alone	That people will observe her confusion Dark, death, evil Insanity	Death Insanity Being murdered
Notes	With insomnia	Her fears cause her to jump out of bed		Hearing becomes very acute
Emotionally	Anxious and restless, becoming frantic, screaming and biting her nails Fear and fright that remain	Anxious and restless, causing her to change place continuously	Sad, wants to go home and doubts that things will improve	Sad and low-spirited Emotional and physical symptoms alternate
Generally	Worse at night Very thirsty Sudden onset of symptoms	Worse after midnight Marked debility Thirsty, drinking little and often Wants to be covered	Chilly, with aversion to open air Sensations of coldness in single parts Perspiration on single parts Lassitude	Trembling, twitching, nervous, shuddering choreic movements

Table 3.3 Fear (Cont'd)

Remedy	Gelsemium	Opium	Phosphorus	Pulsatilla
Occurrence		During labour	Evening/twilight	Evening/twilight
Fears	That her heart will cease to beat unless she is constantly on the move Anticipatory Of falling Death In a crowd	Approach Death Eating Being murdered	When thinking of disagreeable things Being alone in case she dies Death, dark In a crowd During a thunderstrom That something bad will happen	On waking in the morning Dogs, men, ghosts High places Being alone That she is going insane The dark
Notes	Involuntary stools from fright or anticipating an ordeal	Very sensitive hearing		
Emotionally	Hysterical symptoms Irritable, sensitive and excitable	Fear, fright and shock that remain	Imaginative Very anxious and fearful Sensitive to all external impressions	Mild, yielding, apologetic and weepy Changeable
Generally	Trembling Drooping eyelids, red face, cold extremities, hot head Profuse urination	Abnormal absence of pain, secretion, reaction and moral sense	Thirsty for cold drinks Empty feeling in abdomen	Worse warm room Thirstless Desire for fresh air
OTHER REMEDIES	Argentum nitricum; Conium; Ignatia; Rescue remedy			

Table 3.4 *Ill-effects of drugs taken during and/or after labour*

Remedy	Chamomilla	Nux vomica	Opium	Phosphorus	Secale
Effects	Extreme irritability Insomnia	Extreme irritability Insomnia	Depression Drowsy stupor General lack of vital reaction	Vomiting bile	Nausea and vomiting Twitching
Drug taken	Morphine Pethidine	Any	Morphine Pethidine General anaesthetic	General anaesthetic	Syntometrine
Generally	Angry and irritable Tolerates nothing and no-one Snaps and snarls Demands relief, but refuses anything offered	Where general 'de-tox' required Impulsive, quarrelsome and obstinate Knows what she wants and wants it now Dwells on the past	'Spaced-out', dream-like state which she cannot snap out of Drowsy Relives her experiences during the day	'Spaced-out' in euphoric sense Drowsy	Anxious stupor
Worse from	Evening Coffee Fresh air Wind	Morning Coffee Cold wind Uncovering	During sleep Getting up Warmth of bed	Cold During morning During evening	Heat
Better from	Uncovering Perspiring	Heat Lying down Sitting down	Cold Uncovering Constant walking	Good sleep Cold drinks Massage	Cold bathing

OTHER REMEDIES   **Ill-effects of anaesthetic:** Acetic acidum

Table 3.5 *Neonatal respiratory difficulties at delivery*

Remedy	Aconite	Ant tart	Arnica	Arsenicum	Belladonna	Carbo veg	Opium
As if dead	Purplish Blue all over Bradycardia	Pale		Pale but warm		Icy cold Ash pale Bradycardia	Pale
Face	Purple Red Hot	Pale, cold Lower jaw and chin quiver	Hot, body cold	Distorted features, pale	Very red and hot	Pale or cyanotic	Pale
Breath		Gasping for air Throat rattles with mucus	Jerking	Little or no respiratory effort	Anxious Spasmodic	Makes some effort to breathe – wheezing or rattling of mucus	Pale
Asphyxia	Asphyxia	Asphyxia	Asphyxia		Asphyxia		Asphyxia
Cord	Pulsating	Pulsating feebly					Continues to pulsate
Cyanosis						Cyanosis	Cyanosis
Skin		Blue lips and nails		Dry, like parchment			
Spasms				Tetanic with concussion of limbs	Following inability to swallow		Rigid body Tetanic Bending backward
Limbs	Flaccid		Tremble	Stiff, especially feet and knees	Motionless with twitching	Flaccid Limp	
Eyes	Wide open and staring				Pupils dilated Motionless Staring, bloodshot		
NOTES	After precipitate labour With retention of urine	With meconium aspiration	After protracted labour	With or without meconium aspiration		Warmth, stimulants and friction appear to elicit no response	
OTHER REMEDIES	Laurocerasus						

Table 3.6 Pain relief

Remedy	Aconite	Arnica	Belladonna	Caulophyllum	Chamomilla	Cimicifuga	Coffea
Contractions	Very severe In rapid succession Great soreness in the back Parts feel contracted	Distressing Irregular Spasmodic From local sensitiveness Occur on motion of the fetus	Distressing Severe Sudden Spasmodic From nervousness Drawing pain from back to thighs	Distressing Spasmodic Irregular Too short Sharp, cramping pain in uterine ligaments, bladder or groin, flying in all directions, e.g. down legs	Unbearable Spasmodic Tearing in abdomen, shooting down the inner side of the legs Back pain	Severe and distressing Contractions come if the woman is cool and stop when she becomes warmer Tearing, flying around the abdomen with cramping in the hip Spasmodic	Severe and distressing Irregular Worse in the back Spasmodic
Generally	Fearful, restless, moaning Fearful that she or the baby will die With headache and faintness	Denies her suffering Restless Great distress Body feels cold Feels sore all over	Wild, vehement, moaning Wants to escape Face hot, red and flushed Eyes glisten Headache Cramps in legs and hands Faintness Exhaustion	Fretful and exhausted Too weak to develop contractions Fever Thirsty Irritable Trembling Faintness Nausea	Rude, nervous Moaning Tossing about Oversensitive to noise and pain Hot perspiration Faintness Nausea Exhaustion Thirsty Says she can't bear it any more	Talks incessantly, even during contractions Hysterical Complaining Restless Chilly Twitching Trembling Faintness Says she will go crazy	Irritable Excitable Full of ideas Faintness Says she will go crazy
Fears	Can stop the contractions		Fearless			Of death and the delivery	Of death
Birth canal	Os – tender, dry, undilated Cervix – undilated Vulva – dry Vagina – hot, dry, tender, undilating	Uterus fatigued	Os – thin, rigid, hot, tender Cervix – fails to soften, hot and very dry Vagina – hot	Uterus – lack of tone Os – rigid; spasmodic contractions Cervix – needle-like pains Vagina – profuse secretion of mucus	Os – rigid Cervix – fails to soften Vagina – dark coagulated blood	Os – rigid; now dilated, now closed Cervix – fails to soften	Cervix – fails to dilate Vulva – rigid
Hypertension during labour	Hypertension	Hypertension	Hypertension		Hypertension	Hypertension	
Worse from	Noise, including music		Touch, draughts	Cold	Noise and pain	Noise and pain	Draughts
Better from		Being touched	Warmth	Cool fresh air	Cool fresh air		
Type of labour					Protracted		

Table 3.6 Pain relief (Cont'd)

Remedy	Gelsemium	Kali carb	Lycopodium	Nux vomica	Pulsatilla	Secale	Sepia
Contractions	Distressing Cramps in the abdomen go through to the thigh and up the back, then extend to the hips Spasmodic	Distressing Ineffectual Light touch can stop the contractions Sharp bearing-down pain from back to pelvis Cutting in lumbar region Pass down to buttocks Spasmodic	Distressing Spasmodic Going upwards	Severe Irregular Spasmodic drawing in back, descending to thighs Cramps in hand and legs Urge to micturate or defaecate	Distressing Irregular Ineffectual Cutting, pressing Spasmodic in back, appearing suddenly, easing gradually On motion of fetus	Distressing Irregular Ineffectual Sensation of Spasmodic	Severe Spasmodic shooting pains extend upwards Felt in the back weight in the anus
Generally	Chatters during first stage Headache Dark, flushed face Trembling Exhausted even at start of labour Nausea in early labour	Obstinate Oversensitive Restless; chilly after contraction Anxiety felt in the stomach Flatulence Exhaustion	Anxious Weeping Restless Eyes half closed Dictatorial Retention of urine Flatulence	Oversensitive, especially to touch Irritable, nervous, ugly behaviour Trembling Headache Faintness and exhaustion Preterm labour	Changeable, apologetic Wants sympathy Very distressed Face pale Thirstless with dry mouth Faintness Nausea, vomiting Exhaustion Cutting from left to right	Stupor Parts open and loose without action Trembling when contractions cease Refuses to be covered Faintness	Snappy, irritable and indifferent yet resentful if left Cold extremities and flushes of heat Faintness Announces she has had enough
Fears	The delivery	Being alone	Anticipatory	May cause labour			
Birth canal	Uterine inertia Os rigid thick	Cervix fails to soften	Os – spasmodic contractions	Cervix fails to soften, constrictive pain	Uterine inertia Cervix fails to dilate	Uterine inertia Os rigid Cervix fails to soften	Cervix hard Os rigid
Hypertension during labour	Hypertension			Hypertension			Hypertension
Worse from		Light touch	Noise	Draught of fresh air			
Better from	Bending forward; motion	Hard pressure on back	Movement		Fresh air	Fresh air	Crossing the legs
Type of labour			Precipitate	Protracted	Protracted		
NOTES			Finds relief by alternately pressing and relaxing her foot against a support		Finds relief by pressing against the foot of the bed with her feet		

OTHER REMEDIES   Cuprum; Ignatia; Magnesia muriatica; Magnesia phosphorica

Table 3.7 Postpartum haemorrhage

Remedy	Aconite	Belladonna	Bryonia	Carbo veg	Caulophyllum	China
Blood flow	Arterial Bright red Offensive odour	Profuse bleeding Forceful, gushing Coagulates easily Bright red, becoming dark red Feels hot to the woman herself	Profuse bleeding Dark	Passive Continuous Of various appearance	Passive Oozing Dark Profuse bleeding	Passive Intermittent and dark, coagulating easily or: Pale Watery and gushing
Clots		Offensive Dark Large or small				Dark
Cause		Partially adherent placenta			Partially adherent placenta Uterine atony Uterine inertia	Partially adherent placenta Uterine atony
With	Dizziness Fright Fear of death	Downward pressure, as if everything will be forced out Hot red face	Pain in the back Splitting headache Dry mouth and lips Intense thirst Nausea and faintness	Dragging pain Weakness, exhaustion Rapid, weak pulse Difficult breathing No anxiety or restlessness	Tremulous weakness over entire body Exhaustion	Convulsive jerks across abdomen Tinnitus Loss of sight Fainting
Skin				Icy cold Bluish or deathly pale		Cold Blue
NOTES	Worse from motion Bounding pulse	Worse from motion Full, bounding pulse	Worse from slightest movement, even of the foot Worse when speaking	Burning pains, especially across the sacrum and lower part of the spine Wants to be fanned		Dyspnoea Exhaustion Bradycardia Wants to be fanned Intense headache and debility follow
Type of labour		Natural			Precipitate Natural	

Table 3.7 Postpartum haemorrhage (Cont'd)

Remedy	Cinnamomum	Ipecacuanha	Phosphorus	Kali carb	Secale	Sepia
Blood flow	Profuse bleeding Sudden Bright red Passive	Profuse bleeding Gushing Bright red Coagulates quickly	Profuse bleeding Intermittent – pours out freely, then stops for a short time	Clots of coagulated blood	Offensive Passive or gushing Copious Watery, dark or bright red Coagulates easily	Dark Unclotted
Clots					Large	None
Cause		Partially adherent placenta		Partially adherent placenta Uterine atony Atony of blood vessels	Partially adherent placenta Uterine inertia	Chronic congestion of uterus
With	Strain Anaemia Hammering temporal headache	Nausea, faintness and symptoms of collapse Pallor – whiteness of lips and tongue Gasping for breath	Constipation Abdomen sensitive and painful to touch with empty sensation Small of back feels as if broken	Stitching pains Pain begins in the back and extends down over the buttocks	Tingling in hands and constant spreading apart of the fingers Feverish pulse Restless	Darting pains in cervix Sensation of weight in anus Faintness
Skin		Covered in cold perspiration				
NOTES	Primipara – severe flooding after delivery Also secondary postpartum haemorrhage occurring repeatedly during puerperium Worse on any exertion, e.g. overstretching the arms	With cutting pains in the umbilical area	Sensation of heat running up the back Weeping Anxiety Fear	Bounding pulse Especially useful for secondary postpartum haemorrhage occurring one to several weeks after labour	Grande multipara Objective coldness with desire to be uncovered Worse from motion or covering	Rapid emaciation follows Better drawing up the limbs
Type of labour			Difficult		Protracted	

OTHER REMEDIES Acetic acidum; Ferrum; Hamamelis; Sabina; Ustilago. **Secondary postpartum haemorrhage**: Sabina; Ustilago

Because this situation is so acute and life-threatening, there is no time for experiment. If a chosen remedy does not help, conventional medicine must be used

Table 3.8 Retained placenta

Remedy	Belladonna	Caulophyllum	Cimicifuga	Nux vomica	Pulsatilla	Secale	Sepia
Contractions	Hour-glass constriction	Absent	Absent	Hour-glass constriction	Absent or ineffective or Hour-glass constriction	Irregular Hour-glass constriction	Hour-glass constriction
Cause		Uterine atony	Uterine inertia		Uterine inertia Uterine atony. Placenta high up in the fundus	Uterine inertia Uterine atony	Uterine atony
With	Vagina – hot and dry Red face Bloodshot eyes	Exhaustion Weakness	Uterus – tearing pain Headache Pain in eyeballs 'The shakes'	Extreme constrictive pain	Retention of urine Abdomen painful to the touch Continued pain and bleeding	Constant and strong bearing-down sensation Parts feel relaxed	Cervix – sharp, shooting pains
Haemorrhage	Profuse flow of hot blood Coagulates quickly	Passive oozing Dark Profuse Flooding			Intermittent	Dark Passive Watery Copious Offensive	Dark
Generally	Great distress Moaning	Marked weakness, trembling and nervous excitement	Deep sadness Fear of insanity Trembling Alternating symptoms	Very irritable and sensitive to all external stimuli	Mild Tearful Restless Desires air Heat, redness and soreness of epigastrium	Grande multigravida Distressed by pains Desires fresh air but refuses to be covered	Flushes of heat with cold hands and feet
NOTE					Frequently used if there are no clear indications for an alternative remedy		

OTHER REMEDIES Gossypium; Helonias; Ignatia; Sabina

NOTE Arnica may be used as an alternative to syntometrine immediately after the infant is delivered to prevent retained placenta.

Part 4

The puerperium

Table 4.1 After pains

Remedy	Arnica	Caulophyllum	Chamomilla	Cimicifuga
Location		Across lower abdomen, sometimes extending into groins Back and chest		Across lower abdomen extending into groin. Cause flushing of the face
Contractions	Sore/bruised/tearing Violent from bruising and strain on the muscular system	Spasmodic	Distressing Unbearable while breast-feeding Violent and prolonged	Unbearable
With	Flushing of the face Bruising Hypersensitivity of uterine tissues	Muscular weakness Exhaustion	Diarrhoea Lochia profuse, dark and clotted	Nausea and vomiting Uterus does not contract properly Sensitive abdomen
Worse from	During breast-feeding Flatulence		During breast-feeding	Pressure
Better from		Fresh air		
Emotionally	Insists that she is well Fears touch and approach	Nervous	Frantic from pain Ill-natured and spiteful Wants to get away from herself Angry and impossible to please	Low-spirited, cannot tolerate the pain
Generally	Following instrumental delivery Unless contraindicated, a high potency dose of Arnica administered at the end of labour will lessen after-pains	After protracted and exhausting labour Sleepless Weak and exhausted	Thirsty	Oversensitive Restless Sleepless

Table 4.1 After pains (Cont'd)

Remedy	Kali carb	Nux vomica	Pulsatilla	Secale	Silica
Location	Shooting down into hips, buttocks and / or legs	Soreness in uterine region			Hips
Contractions	Stitching Shooting	Violent Protracted	Protracted Changeable – now better, now worse	Frequent, tonic, prolonged, pressing, forcing Unbearable	
With	Backache Perspiration Debility	Scanty, offensive lochia Desire to defaecate	Bad taste in the mouth	Offensive, thin, brown lochia Bearing down Irregular contractions	Trembling of the limbs
Worse from		Fresh air Motion	Towards evening Warm room During breast-feeding	Covering, although she feels cold During breast-feeding	During breast-feeding
Better from	Warmth of bed	Warm room Covered	Fresh air	Cold bathing	
Emotionally	Touchy Angry Irritable Sluggish	Irritable Dreads to be moved or disturbed in any way	Mild Tearful	Anxious stupor	Restless and fidgety Starts from least noise
Generally	Weak and weary	Useful in primipara After protracted labour Wants to be covered Feels faint after every pain	Thirstless Restless Changeable – chill follows heat, particularly when turning over in bed	Grande multiparity Wants to be uncovered The face is very pale	Chilly Cold feeling from nape of neck to vertex

OTHER REMEDIES Cuprum; Hypericum; Magnesia phosphorica; Sabina

Table 4.2 Breast-feeding and breast problems

Remedy	Aconite	Apis	Arnica	Arsenicum	Belladonna	Bryonia
Inadequate lactation	Inadequate lactation	Inadequate lactation		Inadequate lactation	Inadequate lactation	Inadequate lactation
Excessive lactation					Excessive lactation	Excessive lactation
Sore nipples	Cracked	Inverted	Cracked	Cracked Retracted Burning Itching	Acute swelling Burning pain, worse in right breast	Electric-like shocks
Mastitis	Mastitis	Mastitis	Mastitis	Mastitis	Mastitis	Mastitis
Breasts	Hard Tense	Swollen Hard Threatening to ulcerate	Excoriated Ulcerated Violent stitching pains in the middle of left breast	Lump Sensitive to touch	Red streaked from centre to circumference Inflamed Engorged Tender Hot Throbbing Bright red and shiny Swollen	Pale Inflamed Engorged Tender Hot Stony hardness – feel heavy as lead Pain on slightest movement Worse in left breast
With	Possible milk fever and delirium Toothache		Bruised soreness		High fever Dry, burning heat Flushed face Dilated pupils Toothache Headache after breast-feeding	High fever Nausea Extreme thirst Headache after breast-feeding as if her head would burst
Generally/ Emotionally	Fear – says she will die in 24 hours	Jealous Weepy for no reason	Says there is nothing the matter, although this is untrue	Fears to be alone Demanding	Excited Possible delirium Sudden onset	Dryness and thirst Lips begin to crack Irritable when disturbed
Worse from	Night; touch	Heat; touch; 3–5 pm	Touch	After midnight	Jarring	Slightest movement; Cold
Better from	Fresh air	Open air		Heat	Lying down	Alone Supporting the breast
NOTES	To increase/ return flow of milk				May be used to dry up the milk	May be used to dry up the milk after weaning

Table 4.2 Breast-feeding and breast problems (Cont'd)

Remedy	Calcarea carbonica	Causticum	Chamomilla	Graphites	Lycopodium	Phosphorus
Inadequate lactation	Inadequate lactation	Inadequate lactation	Inadequate lactation		Blood instead of milk	Inadequate lactation
Excessive lactation	Excessive lactation		Excessive lactation		Excessive lactation	Excessive lactation
Sore nipples	Hot Swollen Hard	Cracked Herpetic eruption surrounds the nipple	Cracked, tender to touch Inflamed Hot Swollen	Cracked Blistered Swollen	Cracked, bleeding Stinging Burning Itching	Cracked Inflamed Hot Bluish
Mastitis	Mastitis		Mastitis	Mastitis		Mastitis
Breasts	Distended Swollen glands Hot Pains as of excoriation and ulceration of nipples	Burning pains Itching	Hard glands Can hardly bear the pain of breast-feeding	Very sensitive Lymph supply inflamed	Swollen with nodosities Bleeding from ducts and fissures Covered in moist scabs Hot	Swollen Anxious feeling below left breast Burning in the right breast with heat extending to the head Cramping pains
With	Debility Fever Head perspiring at night Watery milk refused by infant Toothache Headache after breast-feeding	Pain extending from the ribs to the left axilla, especially during breast-feeding	Fever Pain in the uterus during breast-feeding Milk is cheesy and contains blood and pus Headache after breast-feeding		Milk without being pregnant	Bitter eructations Increased sexual desire Stitching pains Toothache Headache after breast-feeding
Generally/ Emotionally	Fear that something might happen, e.g. death Chilly	Anxious Oversympathetic	Irritable 'Cannot bear it'	Weeps without cause Timid	Rude Wants company to be in the next room	Wants sympathy; massage Easily reassured
Worse from	Cold air	Twilight	Evening Touch	Night	4–8 pm Touch	Slightest touch
Better From			Uncovering		Fresh air Warm bed	
NOTES	May be used to dry up the milk after weaning		After anger			

Table 4.2 Breast-feeding and breast problems (Cont'd)

Remedy	Phytolacca	Pulsatilla	Sepia	Silica	Staphysagria
Inadequate lactation	Inadequate lactation	Inadequate lactation		Inadequate lactation	
Excessive lactation	Excessive lactation	In those not breast-feeding		Excessive lactation	
Sore nipples	Cracked Swollen, inflamed Sensitive and tender	Cracked Burning Itching	Cracked across crown of nipple Bleeding Seem about to ulcerate	Cracked Bleeding Inverted like a funnel Burning Itching Cutting pain	Cracked
Mastitis	Mastitis	Mastitis		Mastitis	
Breasts	Inflamed Hard – like stone or brick Lumpy, nodular Tender in spots Unbearable pain while breast-feeding starting from the nipple, radiating over the entire body and streaking up and down the spine	Swollen; tense Feel stretched and intensely sore

Pains extend to chest, neck and down the back Pain changes location | Hard Pains shooting; burning | Inflamed Lumpy Deep red in the centre, with rose-coloured periphery Swollen Burning pains worse in left breast; while breast-feeding Pain extends through breast to the shoulder | Pains when milk begins to flow

Breast-feeding almost impossible |
| **With** | Raised temperature – as if 'flu Mammary abscesses and pus Milk with blood Suppressed lochia Bad breath | Thin, watery milk Pain in the uterus while breast-feeding Scanty lochia Milk-white lochia

Headache after breast-feeding | Milk with blood Offensive lochia

Headache after breast-feeding | Cutting pains in uterus Head sweat at night Constipation with no power to expel stool; Back pain High fever Milk with blood refused by infant Headache after breast-feeding | Spasmodic pain in uterus Toothache

Headache after breast-feeding |
Generally/ Emotionally	Unbearable pain Irritable, indifferent and restless	Weeps while breast-feeding	Sad; indifferent to family	Chilly Anxious Excited Yielding	Very irritable Broods over past injuries Feelings suppressed
Worse from		Stuffy atmosphere			Touch
Better from	Supporting the breast	Sympathetic company		Warmth	Warmth
NOTES		Used to dry up the milk when the baby has died or been given up for adoption or after weaning

Also used to restore adequate milk supply which has become deficient following breast infection | | | |

OTHER REMEDIES **Mastitis:** Conium; Lac caninum; Mercurius. **Cracked nipples:** Acetic acidum; Castor equi (if no other symptoms present); Helonias; Hypericum; Rescue remedy cream. **Sore nipples:** Acetic acidum; Castor equi (if no other symptoms present); Mercurius; Rescue remedy cream. **Pain on breast-feeding:** Borax. **Inadequate lactation:** Argentum nitricum; Dulcamara; Ignatia; Urtica urens. **Excessive lactation:** Borax; Conium; Lac caninum; Ustilago.

NOTE Each remedy can be useful for several problems

Table 4.3 Disorders of urinary tract and micturition

Remedy	Aconite	Arnica	Arsenicum	Belladonna	Causticum
Problem	Retention	Incontinence Retention	Incontinence Retention	Incontinence Retention	Incontinence Retention
Cause	Emotional shock Delivery	Difficult/long birth Forceps delivery			
Urging	Frequent, with anxiety	Painful With pressure in bladder	None	Difficult or Continual dribbling	Frequent Passes a little at a time
Pain	Pressing Burning	Soreness	Burning	Shooting in kidney region	
Micturition		Involuntary at night When running Feeble	Burning	Faeces escape during Burning	Expelled slowly Involuntary on cough or sneeze
Urine	Dark Cloudy With red sediment	Pale or brownish-red With brick-coloured sediment	Globules of pus or blood Deep yellow, brownish or greenish	Copious, pale, watery or Turbid, yellow or Red	Scanty, acrid and corrosive or Pale and aqueous
Worse from		Jarring movement Cough	Exertion Coughing	Night	
Better from			Heat		Cold drinks
Emotionally	Anxious and fearful Restless	Averse to being touched Denies her suffering	Anxious Restless Critical Fearful	Excitable Confused Delirious Fierce expression	Pessimistic Suffers pains of others Fights injustice

Table 4.3 Disorders of urinary tract and micturition (Cont'd)

Remedy	Lycopodium	Opium	Secale	Staphysagria
Problem	Retention	Retention	Retention	Retention
Cause		Shock Spasm of sphincter Paralysis of fundus of bladder	Paralysis of bladder after labour	Difficult birth Forceps delivery
Urging	Ineffectual Constant bearing down feeling	None, as from inactivity of the bladder	Continued	Excessively painful emission of urine Frequent
Pain	Severe pain in the back before micturition, which ceases once the flow begins	Absent		Burning
Micturition	Feeble	Feeble stream Slow to start	Drop by drop	Drop by drop
Urine	Clear Transparent With red, sandy sediment	Scanty Bloody Dark brown Brick-dust sediment	Scanty Hot Burning Clear	Scanty, passed drop by drop Deep-coloured
Worse from		Warmth of bed	Heat	Exertion
Better from			Cold bathing	
Emotionally	Weeps before micturition	Dull Confused Apathetic stupor Preceded by exhilaration or delirum	Anxious stupor	Follows a sense of mental or physical assault, where feelings were not expressed at the time

OTHER REMEDIES **Incontinence:** Argentum nitricum; Trillium pendulum. **Retention:** Hypericum.

Table 4.4 Physical trauma

Remedy	Arnica	Bellis perennis	Calendula	Causticum	Chamomilla
After caesarean section **After forceps delivery** **After episiotomy**	Caesarean section Forceps delivery Episiotomy	Caesarean section	Forceps delivery Episiotomy	Episiotomy	Caesarean section
Trauma	Wounds Pain Prevents swelling and bruising of soft tissues	Bumps Lumps Old injuries	Where skin is broken Aids regeneration		
With	Shock Sore/bruised feeling Bad dreams Does not wish to be touched Denies her suffering	Bruised soreness not helped by Arnica Where lump remains	Offensive discharge Pain is more severe than the wound warrants	Pain makes it almost impossible to walk Sadness and fright	Unbearable pain The woman is so sensitive to the pain that she becomes enraged by it Snaps, snarls and demands relief
Worse from				Coffee Change of weather	Evening Fresh air Coffee Wind
Better from				Cold drinks Heat	Uncovering
NOTES	Useful before Hypericum for intense pain *Do not apply externally to broken skin*		Apply externally Alternate with other remedies, e.g. Arnica or Bellis perennis as required. Used with Hypericum as an ingredient in Hypercal tincture. Add 5 drops to a glass of water and apply to wound		

Table 4.4 Physical trauma (Cont'd)

Remedy	Opium	Phosphorus	Secale	Staphysagria
After caesarean section After forceps delivery After episiotomy	Caesarean section	Caesarean section	Caesarean section	Caesarean section Forceps delivery Episiotomy
Trauma	'Spaced-out' feeling after anaesthetic	Wounds that bleed freely with bright red blood, slow to clot Burning pains		Knife wounds Following unpleasant examination
With	'Dream-like' state of fear after operation Recreates images of the shock during waking hours	Need for sympathy Despite being fearful and irritable when tired or upset, she is easily comforted and reassured	A state of stupor with anxiety May be anguish, fear of death or laughing mania	Feeling of humiliation, anger and indignation especially if the operative procedure was more than expected
Worse from	During sleep On getting up Warmth of bed	Cold During evening During morning	Heat	Exertion Fasting Touch Tobacco
Better from		After sleep Massage Cold drinks	Cold bathing	
NOTE				Also useful following catheterization
OTHER REMEDIES	**After caesarean section:** Acetic acidum; Nux vomica. **After episiotomy:** Acetic acidum; Causticum. **After catheterization:** Hypericum; Magnesia phosphorica. **Trauma in general:** Rescue remedy			

Table 4.5 Postnatal depression

Remedy	China	Cimicifuga	Natrum mur	Pulsatilla	Sepia
Possible cause	Loss of fluids	Fear	Suppressed grief Disappointment Anger	Suppressed grief Disappointment Exhaustion Suppressed lochia	Exhaustion
Weeping	At night	Tearful mood With much sighing	Has difficulty crying Cries on her own	Involuntary, constant Causeless When spoken to	Involuntary Causeless
Worse from	Consolation Touch Being examined or looked at	Afternoon During headache	Consolation Sympathy 10–11 am	Evening Stuffy room	Sympathy, consolation Open air On waking, evening
Better from	Writing			Company Sympathy Fresh air	Exercise Being alone, yet may dread to be alone
Also useful during	Pregnancy	Pregnancy Labour	Pregnancy Labour	Pregnancy Labour	
Generally	Exhausted Appetite lost, returning after one mouthful of food	When dejection lifts, may become excitable, talkative and jump from one subject to another Unable to sleep after breast-feeding	Emaciated, while eating well Chilly	Thirstless Desires fresh air	Chilly Perspires easily Restless, moving around continually
Emotionally	Apathetic, sad and loathing life Inclined to sit and do nothing Thinks herself unfortunate and continually harassed by enemies	Much sadness Feels trapped by having to care for the baby	Constantly dwells on past unpleasant events Her moods may alternate from abject despair and loss of interest in life to hilarity with inappropriate laughter	Changeable Mild, yielding, apologetic and weepy Weak memory, absent- minded and finds it difficult to concentrate Afraid that she is going insane Sits immobile in a silent daze Feels forsaken	Indifferent to her baby and loved ones Feels empty and enjoys nothing Fears that she is going insane Hides herself away Feels she must scream or do something desperate

OTHER REMEDIES Conium; Ignatia

Table 4.6 Puerperal mania

Remedy	Arsenicum	Belladonna	Cimicifuga	Lycopodium	Secale
State	Anxious restlessness drives her from place to place	Violent delirium, wildness and biting Rage Hallucinations and fear of imaginary black animals, insects or faces	Deep sadness 'as if enveloped in a dark cloud' Incessant talk, jumping from one subject to another Hatred and envy	Particularly in the early stages, when she behaves in a haughty manner Hysterical – may laugh and cry at the same time	Laughs, claps her hands above her head and seems beside herself Possibly dancing and jumping
Fears	Death Thieves Being alone	Alternate with mania	Death	Men Noise – easily startled by every sound	Death
Feels	That she contaminates everything she touches	That she is dreaming, when she is really awake	That she will become insane	That she would like to run away from her child Indifferent to the child	Anguished – wild with anxiety
With	Marked prostration Wants to be held during mania	May have suicidal thoughts when walking in the open air Red face, large staring eyes and dilated pupils	As mental/emotional activity increases, so her lochia will stop	Possible nymphomania or unreasonable fear of men Confused about everyday things but is rational talking on abstract subjects	Great objective cold-ness, yet refuses to be covered up due to the burning sensation she feels all over the body
Disposition	Selfish – needs to control everyone and everything to gain security Wants to be looked after Thirsty, drinking in sips	She can do it alone – does not need any help from anyone with the baby Feels imprisoned in her own home	Nervous and hysterical	Physical and mental weakness Full of fears, which may be hidden Desires company in the next room Hunger with sudden satiety	Anxious Muscular twitching may begin in the face Grande multiparity
Worse from	After midnight	After noon, 3 pm Touch	Cold	4–8 pm Foods known to cause flatulence	
Better from	Warmth In company	Forenoon Alone		Open air Motion	Being uncovered Cold
OTHER REMEDIES	Cuprum; Zincum				

Table 4.7 Subinvolution and/or abnormal lochia

Remedy	Aconite	Arnica	Belladonna	Bryonia	Calcarea carb	Carbonica veg	Caulophyllum
Subinvolution		Subinvolution	Subinvolution	Subinvolution	Subinvolution	Subinvolution	Subinvolution
Characteristics of the lochia	Offensive, fetid Returning Scanty Suppressed, following cold, fright or vexation	No outstanding features	Flow increases with every contraction Hot Offensive Scanty Suppressed	Copious Offensive, fetid Suppressed from getting cold	Copious Intermittent Milky Prolonged Returning	Offensive	Dark Prolonged Suppressed
Worse from		Physical exertion Touch Pressure	Jarring movement 3 pm	Motion	Exertion Fresh air	Clothing around the abdomen Extremes of temperature	Hot weather
Better from			Lying down	Lying on painful side Cold and warm applications		Rest Being fanned	Pressure
Emotionally	Very fearful, anxious and restless Very sensitive to pain	Fears touch and approach and insists that there is nothing wrong	Excitable Confused Delirious with fierce expression and glistening eyes	Wants to be left alone, becoming very irritable if disturbed	Anxious and slow-thinking Difficulty concentrating	Anxious Indifferent Slow-thinking	Nervous and apprehensive Fretful Easily displeased
Generally	Feels better in the open air	Exhausted Head is hot, with body and extremities cold	Violence Heat Redness Throbbing	Does not wish to be disturbed in any way	Chilly Sour perspiration on single parts, especially the head	Physical weakness and sluggishness	Sleepless Weak Exhausted With internal trembling
NOTE							May be useful for subinvolution following delivery or spontaneous abortion

Table 4.7 *Subinvolution and/or abnormal lochia* (Cont'd)

Remedy	China	Cimicifuga	Opium	Pulsatilla	Secale	Sepia	Staphysagria
Subinvolution	Subinvolution	Subinvolution	Subinvolution	Subinvolution	Subinvolution	Subinvolution	Subinvolution
Characteristics of the lochia	Copious / Offensive, fetid / Prolonged / Suppressed	Suppressed from becoming cold or excited / Thin	Suppressed following fright	Milky / Returns / Scanty / Suppressed	Suddenly becomes dark brown / Offensive, fetid / Suppressed / Prolonged / Thin / Scanty / With prolonged bearing-down pains	Acrid / Offensive, fetid / Prolonged / White	No outstanding features
Worse from	Light touch	Cold and draughts	Warmth	Stuffy atmosphere	Exertion	Becoming heated / Pressure of clothing	Exertion / Touch / Pressure
Better from	Firm pressure	Gentle, continued motion / Warm wraps	Open air	Weeping and sympathetic company		Vigorous exercise	Warmth / Rest
Emotionally	Apathetic	Deep sadness – as if enveloped in a dark cloud / With fear of insanity	Excitable / Confused / Delirious with fierce expression and glistening eyes	Changeable moods	Anxious / In stupor	Sad, weeping, irritable and averse to company, yet dreads to be alone / Indifferent to husband or baby	Suppresses her emotions, especially indignation, which she usually releases in a violent outburst
Generally	Chilliness / Weakness / Faintness / Oversensitive to pain, noise and touch	Trembling / Alternating symptoms	Abnormal absence of pain, reaction and secretion	Thirstless	Grande multiparity	Chilly / Exhausted by the pressure of responsibility	Very sensitive to pain
NOTE		May be useful where subinvolution occurs after spontaneous abortion					

OTHER REMEDIES   **Subinvolution:** Gossypium; Helonias; Sabina; Ustilago. **Intermittent lochia:** Conium. **Prolonged lochia:** Helonias; Sabina; Trillium pendulum; Ustilago. **Suppressed lochia:** Zincum

Part 5

The baby

Table 5.1 Colic

Remedy	Chamomilla	Ipecacuanha	Nux vomica	Secale	Staphysagria
Abdomen	Bloated – flatus collects in several spots. Hard, tense, distended like a drum			Bloated Tight like a drum	
Signs of pain	Baby screams loudly when passing stool Kicks Draws up his legs	Baby does not like to be moved	Baby extremely irritable Frequent straining due to ineffectual urging to defaecate		
Cause	Breast-feeding mother suffering from anger	Breast-feeding mother suffering from anger or frustration	Breast-feeding mother eating spicy food or drinking too much tea, coffee or cola	Syntometrine	Breast-feeding mother suffering from indignation or vexation
With	Diarrhoea with green/yellow stool Sour breath Vomiting bile or curdled milk Red face – one cheek red, other pale Face perspires during feeding, especially on borders of the hair	Empty belching Nausea Vomiting Copious saliva	Much flatulence	Diarrhoea Watery, olive-green stool	
Worse from	Evening	For movement After eating	Morning After eating Coughing During fever Tight clothing		After drinking Touch
Better from	Uncovering After perspiring Being carried		Warmth of bed Hot drinks Passing stool Passing wind	Baby better with nappy off	
Emotionally/ Generally	Angry, tolerates nothing and nobody – howls when denied something it thinks it wants and throws it angrily away once it is offered	Deathly look, with drawn, bluish face and dark-ringed eyes Anxious, capricious and pleased by nothing	Irritable if chilled or tired Startled easily by sudden noise, bright light or touch	Anxious Stupor	Dislikes being touched May throw things
OTHER REMEDIES	Cuprum; Ignatia; Magnesia muriatica; Magnesia phosphorica				

Table 5.2 Constipation

Remedy	Calcarea carbonica	Causticum	Kali carb	Lycopodium	Nux vomica	Opium	Silica
General condition of child	Obstinate when ill Easily startled by sudden noise or being approached too quickly Head perspires freely when feeding	Cries easily and is frightened of the dark or going to bed on his own	Anxious and irritable May moan during sleep	Angry and fearful of strangers or of being alone Kicks and screams after a nap Child seems better when carried about, screams and rolls around with pain	Very chilly May be irritable	Drowsy during the day and sleepless at night Oversensitive to noise	Irritable and worse for consolation Problems assimilating food May refuse mother's milk Head perspires freely during feeding
Stools	Hard at first, which may be followed by diarrhoea Pale, sour-smelling	Soft, despite constipation	Hard Large Pain before stool Unfinished feeling after Soft	Hard Knotty	After passage of stool, rectum does not feel properly emptied	Hard Dry Black	Hard Knotty Large Impacted May slip back when partially expelled
Urging	Ineffectual	Ineffectual	Ineffectual	Ineffectual Flatulence	Much ineffectual urging and straining	Complete absence of urge to stool, sometimes for days at a time	Constant and ineffectual
Anus		Painful					Seems closed by spasms of its muscles
Appetite				Very hungry baby, nursing often		Poor	
Worse from		Passing flatus	2–4 am	4–8 pm	Morning	Heat	Heat
Better from	Being constipated	Sips of cold water	Warmth of bed	Uncovering		Cold things	

Table 5.3 *Discharges from the eye*

Remedy	Aconite	Apis	Arsenicum	Belladonna
Discharge	Profuse lachrymation	Mucus Purulent	Mucus Purulent Acrid lachrymation	Purulent Acrid lachrymation
Eyelids	Hard Swollen Red	Red ringed Swollen Twitching Itching baby continually rubbing eyes	Burning Swollen Twitching Itching Sore	Swollen Twitching
Eyes	Aching Burning Red Sensitive to light Watering profusely	Burning Red Puffy Sore Stinging	Bloodshot Burning Gritty Extremely sensitive to light Oedema around the eyes	Bloodshot Burning Dry Red conjunctiva Sensitive to light Watering Pupils dilated
Worse from	Cold, dry wind Light	Heat Light	Cold Light After midnight	Heat Light
Better from			Warmth of bed Lying down	
Generally/Emotionally	In a state of great fear Restless Anxious	Fidgety Tearful Nervous Irritable	Wants to be carried around briskly	Easy-going when well Obstinate and prone to tantrums when ill

Table 5.3 Discharges from the eye (Cont'd)

Remedy	Bryonia	Calcarea carbonica	Lycopodium	Natrum mur	Pulsatilla
Discharge	Mucus Purulent	Mucus Purulent Acrid Yellow	Thick mucus Purulent Acrid	Mucus Lachrymation Burning Acrid	Mucus Purulent Offensive Thick Yellow
Eyelids	Swollen	Glued together Swollen Twitching Itching Sore	Glued together Swollen Twitching and itching Ulcerated Red	Heavy Swollen Twitching Sore Especially affecting the right eye	Glued together Swollen Twitching and itching Red Especially affecting the left eye
Eyes	Dry Sore	Gritty Sensitive to light Watering	Sensitive to light Watering	Burning Gritty Sensitive to light	Aching Burning Itching Watering
Worse from	Moving the eyes Touch	Cold Light	Warm applications Light	Exposure to sun Light	Evening Warm room
Better from		Heat Lying down			Cold Cold bathing Fresh air
Generally/ Emotionally	Does not like to be moved Capricious	Happy when well Lethargic and obstinate when ill	May sleep well at night and cry all day	Serious Dislikes too much physical contact	Wants to be carried around gently Clingy and dependent
OTHER REMEDIES	Argentum nitricum; Mercurius; Zincum				

Table 5.4 Minor skin injuries

Remedy	Arnica	Bellis perennis	Sulphuricum acidum
Bruises	With swelling Without discoloration If given early enough, the bruise will not materialize	Bruise has disappeared, leaving a lump or bump	Bluish-black Slow to heal
Worse from	Least touch Motion	Cold bathing	Heat Evening Mid-morning
Better from	Lying down With head low		
NOTES	Promotes healing Controls bleeding Prevents pus formation *Do not apply externally to broken skin*	Useful where Arnica has cleared up the bruising but where a deeper-acting remedy is required After surgery	Useful where Arnica has failed to clear up the bruise Generally: Anaemic Chilly Irritable *This remedy is described more fully in the Appendix*

Table 5.5 Neonatal jaundice

Remedy	Aconite	Arsenicum	Bryonia	Chamomilla	Chelidonium
General condition of child	May be fine on going to bed, but wakens around midnight Resents interference Sudden onset	Wants to be carried around briskly Burning pains, better for warmth	Likes to be carried, though not moved around too much Capricious	Spiteful, whining, screaming and hitting Insists on being carried Cries loudly when held still or put down Capricious	Marked lethargy The yellowness of the face is especially marked on the nose and cheeks
Predisposing factor					
Skin		Dry Rough Scaly	Yellow Hot Painful	Yellow colour over whole body	Cold Clammy Yellow Itching
With	Intense thirst Yellow sclera	Photophobia Yellow sclera Yellow face	Yellow face	Contracted pupils Yellow sclera	Contracted pupils Dirty yellow sclera Profuse lachrymation Yellow tongue One foot is cold while the other is hot
Worse from	Night Warm room	3 am Cold Damp	Any motion	Evening Fresh air	Motion Touch 4 am and 4 pm Lying on right side
Better from	Fresh air	Heat Lying down	Fresh air Firm pressure	Uncovering	Pressure Bending backwards Feeding gives temporary relief
NOTE					This is the MAIN REMEDY FOR JAUNDICE IN BABIES. Frequently used when there are no clear indications for another remedy

Table 5.5 Neonatal jaundice (Cont'd)

Remedy	China	Nux vomica	Phosphorus	Sepia
General condition of child	Sensitive Dislikes being examined Irritable and mischievous in the morning Very weak	Irritable if chilled, tired or overfed Constipated Possible fainting	When healthy, lively, affectionate, excitable When ill, becomes irritable and apathetic Desires touch and affection	Chilly, sweating easily and profusely Smells sour Does not wish to be touched Yellowness more marked across saddle of nose Dark rings under the eyes
Predisposing factor	Loss of vital fluids			
Skin	Yellow Sore – made worse by light touch but better by firm pressure	Pale yellow	Yellow with yellow spots	Yellow Chapped with deep cracks
With	Yellow sclera Thirsty Appetite only when feeding Yellow face Thick yellow coating on the tongue One hand icy cold while the other is warm	Yellow sclera, principally in lower part of eyeballs Dislike for food Yellow face	Yellowish sclera	Yellow sclera Drooping eyelids Vomits after eating Yellow face
Worse from	Open air After feeding	Morning Cold	Cold Change of weather	Damp After sweating
Better from	Hard pressure	After nap Strong pressure	After sleep Cold drink Massage	Pressure Hot applications Cold bathing After sleep

OTHER REMEDIES Magnesia muriatica; Mercurius

Table 5.6 *Oral and rectal candidiasis*

Remedy	Antimonium-tart	Arsenicum	Calcarea carbonica	Natrum mur
Thrush	Accompanied by forcible vomiting of milk, followed by exhaustion and sleep	Especially on the tongue Accompanied by merasmus Profound prostration Low fever, ulceration Possible diarrhoea	Especially on roof of mouth Accompanied by vomiting of milk in sour cakes or curds	Especially on the tongue and gums Accompanied by herpetic eruption around lips Increased salivation
General condition of child	The child wants to be carried, but not touched-clings to the person carrying him and cries or whines if anyone touches him	Restless In constant distress The skin may be harsh, dry and tawny	Happy when well Lethargic and obstinate when ill Flabby, feeble and tired The stomach may be distended, even when the rest of the body is emaciated	Serious Dislikes too much physical contact The baby has a voracious appetite, yet suffers from emaciation, especially of the upper part of the body
Worse from	Warmth Lying down Touch	1–2 am Cold	Cold	Consolation
Better from	Cool air Uncovering Motion	Warmth In company	Heat Lying down	Heat in general
OTHER REMEDIES	Borax; Mercurius; Sulphuricum acidum			

Table 5.7 Sleeplessness

Remedy	Aconite	Belladonna	Chamomilla	Phosphorus	Pulsatilla
Sleeplessness	With fear and excitement Tosses about in agony	Restless Twitching during sleep	Attacks of anguish at night	Wakeful Restless at night	With twitching arms and legs
Cause	Fear or fright		Anger, pain, stimulants	Strong emotions	Cold
With sleepiness		Yet is unable to sleep	During the day	After feeding Sleepy at 7 pm	In afternoon and evening
Sleep	Light Restless With startings	Troubled	Snoring Starts with fright during sleep Limbs twitch on falling asleep	Unrefreshing Cries during sleep	Irregular Restless Cries during sleep
Position	Unable to sleep on the side Lies on back with one hand under the head		Yawning and stretching	Unable to sleep on back or left side	Lies on back with knees raised and arms placed over head and feet poking out from under the covers
Waking	Frequent	Frequent as if from fright	Frequent	Frequent Feels too hot 4 am	Frequent Confused on waking Waking as if from fright
Worse from	Around midnight (before or after)	Around midnight (before or after)	At night Between midnight and 2 am	At night Before midnight and again after 4 am	Before midnight until 2 am
Generally	Anxious May wake around midnight with some physical complaint	Face is hot and red Swallowing is impeded	Cries loudly when held still or put down Wants to be rocked Hits parents, whines, screams and cannot be comforted	Lively, affectionate and excitable when healthy Irritable and impatient when unwell Wants to be stroked and touched	Whining, tearful infant, wants to be carried around gently

Part 6

Materia medica – remedy pictures (main remedies)

Remedy abbreviations for suggested uses in the Materia Medica are explained in Appendix 2.

Aconite (Acon) *Aconitum napellus*. Other names: Monkshood, Helmet flower

---

Prime indications:
- **Great fear of death**
- **Extreme anxiety**
- **Agonized restlessness**
- **Painful inflammation**
- **Numbness and tingling**
- **High fever with dry skin**
- **Rapid bounding pulse**

Additional characteristics:
General
- Suited to people of robust constitution
- Complaints come on suddenly

Emotional
- Irritability
- Sensitivity to pain
- Delirium

Caused by
- Exposure to cold dry winds
- Fright, anger, shock
- Getting chilled while perspiring

Sensations
- Prickling
- Enlargement of parts
- Heat of affected parts
- General coldness

Pains
- Cutting
- Stitching
- Burning

Worse
- Night
- Noise (including music)
- Rising up in bed
- Violent emotions
- Being chilled
- From drinking cold water
- Lying on affected side
- Light
- Being jolted

Better
- Open air
- Warm perspiration
- Repose

Note Aconite is followed well by Arnica, Arsenicum or Bryonia.

Suggested uses:
- Discharges from the eye[9]* (Apis; Arg-n; Ars; Bell; Bry; Calc; Lyc; Nat-m; Merc; Puls; Zinc)
- Failure to progress[6,13] (Arn; Bell; Bor; Carb-v; Caul; Cham; Chin; Cimic; Cinn; Coff; Cupr; Gels; Ign; Kali-c; Kali-p; Lyc; Mag-m; Nat-m; Nux-v; Op; Puls; Sec; Sep)
- Fear during pregnancy, labour and after delivery, i.e. that she or the baby will die[1,3,4,5,6,8,9,11,13] (Arg-n; Ars; Calc; Cimic; Gels; Ign; Op; Phos; Puls; Rescue remedy)
- Haemorrhoids[6] (Ars; Collins; Ham; Hyp; Ign; Kali-c; Lyc; Nat-m; Nux-v; Puls; Sep; Staph)
- Hypertension during labour[2] (Arn; Apis; Bell; Cham; Cimic; Gels; Ign; Merc; Nat-m; Op; Puls; Sep)
- Inadequate lactation[2,9] (Arg-n; Ars; Apis; Bell; Bry; Calc; Caust; Cham; Dulc; Graph; Ign; Lyc; Phos; Phyt; Puls; Sil; Urt-u)
- Insomnia in mother[2,3,4,6,8] (Bell; Bellis-p; Coff; Con; Gels; Ign; Kali-c; Nux-v; Op; Puls)
- Labour at standstill[13] (Carb-v; Chin; Cimic; Cinn-m; Gels; Nux-v; Op)
- Mastitis[9] (Apis; Arn; Ars; Bell; Bry; Cham; Con; Graph; Lac-c; Lyc; Merc; Phos; Phyt; Puls; Sil)
- Neonatal jaundice[7,8,9,10] (Ars; Bry; Cham; Chel; Chin; Mag-m; Merc; Nux-v; Phos; Sep)
- Neonatal respiratory difficulties at delivery[13] (Ant-t; Arn; Ars; Bell; Carb-v; Laur; Op)
- Pain relief during labour[12] (Arn; Bell; Caul; Cham; Cimic; Coff; Cupr; Gels; Ign; Kali-c; Lyc; Mag-m; Mag-p; Nux-v; Puls; Sec; Sep)
- Postpartum haemorrhage[3,4,6,8,13] (Acet-ac; Bell; Bry; Carb-v; Caul; Chin; Cinn-m; Ferr; Ham; Kali-c; Phos; Sab; Sec; Sep; Ust)
- Pruritus vulvae[2,9] (Ars; Bell; Bor; Calc; Coff; Collins; Graph; Ham; Helon; Lyc; Merc; Sep)
- Retention of urine after labour[4,6] (Arn; Ars; Bell; Caust; Hyp; Lyc; Op; Sec; Staph)
- Shock (emotional)[3,4,8,13] (Acet-ac; Arn; Hyp; Ign; Op; Phos; Rescue remedy; Staph)
- Sleeplessness in infant (Bell; Cham; Phos; Puls)
- Sore, cracked nipples[2] (Acet-ac; Arn; Ars; Bell; Calc; Cast-eq; Caust; Cham; Graph; Hyp; Lac-c; Lyc; Merc; Phos; Phyt; Puls; Sep; Sil; Staph; Rescue remedy)
- Spontaneous abortion[2,5,6,8,9,10,13] (Alet; Apis; Arn; Bell; Caul; Cimic; Ferr; Goss; Helon; Ip; Kali-c; Kali-p; Nux-v; Op; Puls; Sab; Sec; Sep; Tril)
- Vaginal bleeding during pregnancy[13] (Arn; Bell; Caul; Ign; Op; Puls; Sab; Sec; Sep; Tril)

---

*References in the Materia Media appear on p. 132.

Antimonium tartaricum (Ant-t). Other names: Potassium antimony tartarate, $2[K(SbO)C_4H_4O_6]H_2O$, tartar emetic

Prime indications:[7]
- **Coarse rattling of mucus in the chest, with scanty expectoration**
- **Nausea coming in waves, better vomiting**
- **Aversion to being touched or looked at**
- **Prostration, faintness, drowsiness, coldness**
- **Thirstlessness during fever, otherwise great thirst**
- **Worse from warmth and from cold or damp air**

Additional characteristics:
General
- Torpid and phlegmatic
- Lacking in vital energy
- Increased discharges from mucous membranes
- Trembling, twitching, convulsions

Emotional
- Irritable – averse to being looked at or touched
- Anxious and restless
- Apathetic, drowsy and dull
- Wants to be left alone

Caused by
- Damp living conditions
- Getting chilled
- Suppression of eruptions

Worse
- Evening
- Night
- From anger
- Warmth, warm bed, warm weather
- Cold wet weather or air
- Eating
- After vomiting
- Lying down
- Touch

Better
- Cool air
- Uncovering
- Motion

Note Antimonium tartaricum follows Silica or Pulsatilla well.

Suggested uses:
- Candida (oral) in infants[5,6] (Ars; Bor; Calc; Nat-m; Merc; Sul-ac) with vomiting of milk
- Nausea[3,7,12] (Acet-ac; Alet; Ars; Chel; Goss; Ip; Nux-v; Phos; Puls; Sep) with frequent vomiting of bitter, sour

substances, accompanied by weakness, cold sweat and anxiety
- Neonatal respiratory difficulties at delivery[3,6,7,8,12,13] (Acon; Arn; Ars; Bell; Carb-v; Cupr; Laur; Op) where infant is pale, breathless and gasping. Relieves the death rattle

Apis (Apis) *Apis mellifica*. Other names: Honey bee

Prime indications
- **Burning, stinging pains**
- **Thirstless, even with burning heat**
- **Prostration**
- **Scanty or suppressed urine**
- **Oedematous swellings**
- **Urticaria**

Additional characteristics:
General
- Fidgety
- Tearful
- Nervous
- Irritable
- Drowsiness
- Coma

Emotional
- Excitable, in spite of weakness
- Hysterical
- Fickle
- Jealous

Sensations
- Bruised soreness
- Tightness (chest, abdomen, oedema, limbs)

Worse
- Warmth
- Pressure
- Lying down
- Afternoon, 3 pm
- Motion

Better
- Cold
- Cold applications
- Change of position

Note Apis is followed well by Arnica, Arsenicum or Pulsatilla[12]

Suggested uses:
- Carpal tunnel syndrome[1,8] (Ars; Calc; Caust; Lyc; Sep)
- Eye discharges in infants[8,9] (Acon; Arg-n; Ars; Bell; Bry; Calc; Lyc; Nat-m; Puls) of mucus or pus
- Gestational hypertension[3,6,9,12] (Acet-ac; Ars; Bell; Calc;

Ferr; Gels; Helon; Kali-c; Lyc; Merc; Nat-m; Op; Phos; Puls; Sep; Zinc)
- Hypertension during labour (Acon; Bell; Cham; Cimic; Gels; Ign; Merc; Nat-m; Op; Puls; Sep)
- Inadequate lactation[8,9] (Acon; Arg-n; Ars; Bell; Bry; Calc; Caust; Cham; Dulc; Graph; Ign; Lyc; Phos; Phyt; Puls; Sil; Urt-u)
- Mastitis[9,10] (Acon; Arn; Ars; Bell; Bry; Calc; Cham; Con; Graph; Lac-c; Lyc; Merc; Phos; Phyt; Puls; Sil)
- Nappy rash where skin is red, shiny, hot and sore
- Proteinuria[2,3,4,8,9,12] (Ars; Bell; Ferr; Gels; Helon; Kali-c; Lyc; Merc; Nat-m; Phos; Sab; Sep)
- Spontaneous abortion[1,3,8,9,11] (Acon; Alet; Arn; Bell; Caul; Cimic; Ferr; Goss; Helon; Ip; Kali-c; Kali-p; Nux-v; Op; Sab; Sec; Sep; Tril). Tendency to abortion between 4 and 16 weeks
- Suppressed urine – proteinuria or containing casts

Arnica (Arn) *Arnica montana.* Other names: Leopard's bane, fall-kraut, mountain tobacco, sneezewort

---

Prime indications:[7]
- **Trauma**
- **Injuries to soft tissues**
- **Haemorrhage**
- **Bruising**
- **Stupor, but answers correctly**
- **Painful eruptions**
- **Head hot, with body and extremities cold**

Additional characteristics:
General
- Oversensitive – cannot bear the pain
- Startles easily
- Exhausted and tired
- Sleepless before and after midnight
- Wakes terrified
- Painful glands
- Restless

Emotional
- Fears touch and approach
- Insists all is well
- Irritable
- Forgetful
- Apathetic
- Indifferent
- Confused
- Despairing and depressed

Caused by
- Injury
- Overexertion

Sensations
- Sore/bruised, better for changing position
- Knotted
- Bed feels too hard

Pains
- Aching
- Pressing
- Tearing
- Stitching
- Burning
- Numbness

Worse
- Evening
- Night
- Touch
- Pressure
- Physical exertion
- During and after sleep
- Noise

Better
- Lying down
- Open air
- Heat

Notes
- Arnica follows well after Aconite, Apis, Hamamelis or Ipecacuanha
- Arnica is followed well by Aconite, Arsenicum, Bryonia, Ipecacuanha or Sulphuric acid
- Encourages expulsion of the placenta, if given immediately after the baby is delivered. It will also help prevent haemorrhage, after-pains when the baby sucks and septic condition

Suggested uses:
- Abdominal pain during pregnancy due to activity of fetus[7,8,9,13] (Acet-ac; Ars; Cupr; Nux-v; Puls; Sep; Staph)
- After-pains[2,3,6,7,8,9,11,13] (Caul; Cham; Cimic; Cupr; Hyp; Kali-c; Mag p; Nux-v; Puls; Sab; Sec; Sil), worse when nursing[13]
- Bruising[6,8] (Bell-p; Sul-ac)
- Failure to progress[6,7,9,13] (Acon; Bell; Bor; Carb-v; Caul; Cham; Chin; Cimic; Cinn-m; Coff; Cupr; Gels; Ign; Kali-c; Kali-p; Lyc; Mag-m; Nat-m; Nux-v; Op; Puls; Sec; Sep)
- Hypertension during labour (Acon; Apis; Bell; Cham; Cimic; Gels; Ign; Merc; Nat-m; Op; Puls; Sep)
- Incontinence[7,8,9,11,12] (Arg-n; Ars; Bell; Caust; Tril)
- Ligament pain/sciatica[8] (Bell-p; Caust; Ferr; Mag-p; Phyt; Puls; Sep)
- Mastitis[6,9] (Acon; Apis; Ars; Bell; Bry; Calc; Cham; Con; Graph; Lac-c; Lyc; Merc; Phos; Phyt; Puls; Sil)

- Neonatal respiratory difficulties at delivery[8,13] (Acon; Ant-t; Ars; Bell; Carb-v; Laur; Op)
- Pain relief during labour (Acon; Bell; Caul; Cham; Cimic; Coff; Cupr; Gels; Ign; Kali-c; Lyc; Mag-m; Mag-p; Nux-v; Puls; Sec; Sep)
- Phlebitis (Bry; Ham; Puls)
- Postpartum bruising, ache and soreness[3,10] (Bell-p; Calen; Caust; Cham; Hyp; Nux-v; Op; Phos; Sec; Staph)
- Retained placenta, prevention of[2,5,12] (Bell-p)
- Retention of urine[3,6,7,12,13] (Acon; Ars; Bell; Caust; Hyp; Lyc; Op; Sec; Staph)
- Shock[6] (emotional) and trauma after a difficult labour, e.g. precipitate labour or following caesarean or instrumental delivery[3,4,8,12,13] (Acet-ac; Acon; Hyp; Ign; Op; Phos; Rescue remedy; Staph)
- Sore, cracked nipples[3,6,9] (Acet-ac; Acon; Ars; Bell; Calc; Cast-eq; Caust; Cham; Graph; Hyp; Lac-c; Lyc; Merc; Phos; Phyt; Puls; Sep; Sil; Staph; Rescue remedy)
- Spontaneous abortion[2,5,6,8,9,12,13] (Acon; Alet; Apis; Bell; Caul; Cimic; Ferr; Goss; Helon; Ip; Kali-c; Kali-p; Nux-v; Op; Puls; Sab; Sec; Tril), following an accident
- Subinvolution[3] (Bell; Bry; Calc; Carb-v; Caul; Chin; Cimic; Goss; Helon; Op; Puls; Sab; Sec; Sep; Staph; Ust)
- Vaginal bleeding during pregnancy (Acon; Bell; Caul; Ign; Kali-c; Op; Puls; Sab; Sec; Sep; Tril)

Arsenicum (Ars) *Arsenicum album*. Other names: Arsenious trioxide As_2O_3

Prime indications:[7]
- **Anxiety, restlessness**
- **Fear of death**
- **Burning pains, made better by heat and worse by cold**
- **Marked faintness, prostration**
- **Itching, burning skin eruptions**
- **Worse after midnight**
- **Lack of vital heat**
- **Thirsty, drinking little and often**

Additional characteristics:
General
- Trembling, twitching and jerking
- Emaciation of affected parts
- Acrid, scanty, offensive discharges

Emotional
- Selfish, needing to control everyone around them to gain a sense of security
- Fear of being alone
- Suspicious
- Impatient
- Irritable

Caused by
- Eating food that has 'gone bad'
- Cold food and ice water
- Abuse of tobacco or alcohol

Pains
- Burning
- Like hot needles or wires
- Dryness of internal and external parts

Worse
- After midnight, 1–2 am
- Twilight
- Night
- Cold or becoming cold
- Cold food or drink
- Lying down
- Physical exertion
- Climbing stairs
- After eating
- After alcohol
- 1 pm[4]

Better
- Daytime
- Evening
- Open air
- Warm food or drink
- Hot applications
- Rising up or sitting
- In company

Notes
- Arsenicum follows Aconite, Apis, Arnica, Belladonna, Chamomilla, China or Ipecacuanha well[7]
- Arsenicum is followed well by Nux vomica

Suggested uses:
- Abdominal pain during pregnancy[8,9] (Acet-ac; Arn; Cupr; Nux-v; Puls; Sep; Staph) due to motion of the fetus
- Anaemia[6,7,11] (Alet; Calc; Carb-v; Chin; Cupr; Ferr; Helon; Kali-c; Kali-p; Merc; Nat-m; Phos; Puls; Sep; Staph; Sul-ac; Tril)
- Candida[1,5,6,8,11] in infants (Ant-t; Bor; Calc; Nat-m; Merc; Sul-ac)
- Carpal tunnel syndrome[1,8] (Apis; Calc; Caust; Lyc; Sep)
- Cystitis[6] (Acon; Apis; Caust; Lyc; Merc; Nux-v; Puls; Sep; Staph)
- Diarrhoea[7,12] (Chin; Merc; Phos; Puls)
- Dizziness and fainting during pregnancy[6,8,9] (Bell; Cimic; Gels; Ign; Kali-c; Laur; Nat-m; Nux-v; Puls; Sep)
- Eye discharges in infants[6,8] (Acon; Apis; Arg-n; Bell; Bry; Calc; Lyc; Merc; Nat-m; Puls; Zinc) of mucus or pus

- Fear[1,7,12] (Acon; Arg-n; Calc; Cimic; Gels; Ign; Op; Phos; Puls; Rescue remedy) during labour[8]
- Frequency of micturition[8] (Bell; Caust; Nat-m; Puls; Sep)
- Gestational hypertension[3,6,9] (Acet-ac; Apis; Bell; Calc; Ferr; Gels; Helon; Kali-c; Lyc; Merc; Nat-m; Op; Phos; Puls; Sep; Zinc)
- Haemorrhoids[1,2,8,10,11] (Collins; Ham; Hyp; Ign; Kali-c; Lyc; Nat-m; Nux-v; Puls; Sab; Sep; Staph)
- Inadequate lactation (Acon; Arg-n; Apis; Bell; Bry; Calc; Caust; Dulc; Graph; Ign; Lyc; Phyt; Puls; Sil; Urt-u)
- Incontinence[8] (Arg-n; Arn; Bell; Caust; Tril)
- Mastitis (Acon; Apis; Arn; Bell; Bry; Calc; Cham; Con; Graph; Lac-c; Lyc; Merc; Phos; Phyt; Puls; Sil)
- Nausea and vomiting[2,3,5,6,7,8,9,12] (Acet-ac; Alet; Chel; Goss; Ip; Nux-v; Phos; Puls; Sep)
- Neonatal jaundice[3,6,11] (Acon; Bry; Cham; Chel; Chin; Mag-m; Merc; Nux-v; Phos; Sep)
- Neonatal respiratory difficulties at delivery[13] (Acon; Ant-t; Arn; Bell; Carb-v; Laur; Op)
- Proteinuria[2,3,4,8,9,11,12] (Apis; Bell; Ferr; Gels; Helon; Kali-c; Lyc; Merc; Nat-m; Phos; Sab; Sep)
- Pruritus vulvae[9] (Acon; Bor; Calc; Coff; Collins; Graph; Ham; Helon; Lyc; Merc; Sep; Sil)
- Puerperal mania (Bell; Cimic; Cupr; Lyc; Sec; Zinc)
- Retention of urine after labour[6,3,7,9,13] (Acon; Arn; Bell; Caust; Hyp; Lyc; Op; Sec; Staph)
- Sore, cracked nipples[2] (Acet-ac; Acon; Arn; Bell; Calc; Cast-eq; Caust; Cham; Graph; Hyp; Lac-c; Lyc; Merc; Phos; Phyt; Puls; Sep; Sil; Staph; Rescue remedy)

Belladonna (Bell) *Atropa belladonna*. Other names: Deadly nightshade, common dwale, sorcerer's cherry, witch's berry

---

Prime indications:[7]
- **Sudden violent onset**
- **Congestion**
- **Redness**
- **Burning heat, high fever**
- **Pulsation**
- **Sensitive to touch, light**
- **Twitching of muscles, convulsions**
- **Overexcitement and sensibility of all the nerves**

Additional characteristics:
General
- Starting
- Jerking
- Spasms
- Constriction of hollow organs, orifices
- Perspiration only on covered parts
- Discharges hot and scanty

- Mucous membranes dry
- Pulse rapid, full and bounding
- Wild look

Emotional
- Nervous and sensitive
- Lively and entertaining when well but violent when ill
- Irritable
- Restless
- Fearful
- Wild delirium
- Hallucinations
- Biting rage

Sensations
- Heaviness
- Feeling 'full'
- Of ball in internal parts
- Of band around the part

Pains
- Throbbing
- Stitching, cutting or stabbing
- Come and go quickly

Worse
- Afternoon, 3 pm
- Night
- Cold draughts / open air
- Bright light
- Touch, jar, motion
- Lying on affected side
- Letting affected part hang down

Better
- Forenoon
- Warmth
- Lying down
- Sitting
- Bending backwards

Notes
- Belladonna follows Cuprum, Mercurius or Phosphorus well
- Belladonna is followed well by Arsenicum, Calcarea carbonica, Chamomilla, China, Conium or Silica

Suggested uses:
- Backache during pregnancy[3,8,11,12] (Bry; Calc; Cimic; Ferr; Hyp; Kali-c; Kali-p; Lyc; Nat-m; Nux-v; Phos; Puls; Sep; Sil; Zinc)
- Dizziness and fainting during pregnancy[2,5,6,8,9] (Ars; Cimic; Gels; Ign; Kali-c; Laur; Nat-m; Nux-v; Puls; Sep) due to postural hypotension
- Excessive lactation[2,3,9] (Bor; Bry; Calc; Cham; Con; Lac-c; Lyc; Phos; Phyt; Ust)

- Eye discharges in infants[6,9] (Acon; Apis; Arg-n; Ars; Bry; Calc; Lyc; Nat-m; Puls; Zinc)
- Failure to progress[3,7,9,12] (Acon; Arn; Bor; Carb-v; Caul; Cham; Chin; Cimic; Cinn-m; Coff; Cupr; Gels; Ign; Kali-c; Kali-p; Lyc; Mag-m; Nat-m; Nux-v; Op; Puls; Sec; Sep)
- Frequency of micturition[5,8] (Ars; Caust; Nat-m; Puls; Sep)
- Gestational hypertension[3] (Acet-ac; Apis; Ars; Calc; Ferr; Gels; Helon; Kali-c; Lyc; Merc; Nat-m; Op; Phos; Puls; Sep; Zinc)
- Hypertension during labour[2] (Acon; Apis; Arn; Cham; Cimic; Gels; Ign; Merc; Nat-m; Op; Puls; Sep)
- Inadequate lactation[8,9] (Acon; Arg-n; Ars; Apis; Bry; Calc; Caust; Cham; Dulc; Graph; Ign; Lyc; Phos; Phyt; Puls; Sil; Urt-u)
- Incontinence[8,11,12] (Arg-n; Arn; Ars; Caust; Tril)
- Insomnia[3,4,6,8,12] during pregnancy (Acon; Bell-p; Coff; Gels; Kali-c; Nux-v; Op; Puls)
- Mastitis[1,4,6,7,9,11,12] (Acon; Apis; Arn; Ars; Bry; Cham; Con; Graph; Lac-c; Lyc; Merc; Phyt; Puls; Sil), smooth redness radiates in streaks to surrounding parts
- Neonatal respiratory difficulties at delivery[7,8,13] (Acon; Ant-t; Arn; Ars; Carb-v; Laur; Op)
- Pain relief during labour[12] (Acon; Arn; Caul; Cham; Cimic; Coff; Cupr; Gels; Ign; Kali-c; Lyc; Mag-m; Mag-p; Nux-v; Puls; Sec; Sep)
- Postpartum haemorrhage[2,3,4,7,8,11,12,13] (Acet-ac; Acon; Bry; Carb-v; Caul; China; Cinn-m; Ferr; Ham; Ip; Kali-c; Phos; Sab; Sec; Sep; Ust)
- Proteinuria[9] (Apis; Ars; Ferr; Gels; Helon; Kali-c; Lyc; Merc; Nat-m; Phos; Sab; Sep)
- Pruritus vulvae[6,9] (Acon; Ars; Bor; Calc; Coff; Collins; Graph; Helon; Lyc; Merc; Sep; Sil)
- Puerperal mania[2,3,5,6,7] (Ars; Cimic; Cupr; Lyc; Sec; Zinc)
- Respiratory difficulties in the newborn[13] (Acon; Ant-t; Arn; Ars; Carb-v; Cupr; Laur; Op)
- Retained placenta[8,9,13] (Caul; Cimic; Goss; Ign; Nux-v; Puls; Sab; Sec; Sep)
- Retention of urine[11] (Acon; Arn; Ars; Caust; Hyp; Lyc; Op; Sec; Staph)
- Sleeplessness in infant[4,9] (Acon; Cham; Phos; Puls)
- Sore, cracked nipples[1] (Acet-ac; Acon; Arn; Ars; Calc; Cast-eq; Caust; Cham; Graph; Hyp; Lac-c; Lyc; Merc; Phos; Phyt; Puls; Sep; Sil; Staph; Rescue remedy)
- Spontaneous abortion[2,3,8,9,13] (Acon; Alet; Apis; Arn; Caul; Cimic; Ferr; Goss; Helon; Ip; Kali-c; Kali-p; Nux-v; Op; Puls; Sab; Sec; Sep; Tril) between 12–16 weeks
- Subinvolution[8] (Arn; Bry; Calc; Carb-v; Caul; Chin; Cimic; Goss; Helon; Op; Puls; Sab; Sec; Sep; Staph; Ust)
- Vaginal bleeding during pregnancy[12] (Acon; Arn; Caul; Ign; Kali-c; Op; Puls; Sab; Sec; Sep; Tril)

Bellis (Bell-p) *Bellis perennis*. Other names: Garden daisy, English daisy, bruisewort

Prime indications:
- **Relief of bruised soreness after childbirth where Arnica has failed**
- **Where Arnica has cleared bruising, but a lump remains**
- **Illness following chilling when overheated**

Additional characteristics:
General
- Marked action on engorged uterus and breasts
- Slight giddiness
- Loss of appetite
- Nausea

Caused by
- Accident / injury
- Surgery
- Getting wet when overheated
- Drinking cold drinks when overheated

Worse
- Injury
- Touch
- Becoming chilled when hot

Better
- Continued motion

Note Bellis follows Arnica well in bruising

Suggested uses:
- After caesarean (Acet-ac; Arn; Cham; Hyp; Nux-v; Op; Phos; Sec; Staph)
- Abdominal pain during pregnancy (Acet-ac; Ars; Bry; Cimic; Cupr; Puls) due to uterine ligament tension; of sudden onset, with sore uterus and stiffness in the lower abdomen
- Bruising (Arn; Sul-ac)
- Inability to walk during pregnancy[2] from straining abdominal muscles, internal bruising of the uterus due to fetal activity or mechanical pressure on the groins
- Insomnia[5,6] (Acon; Bell; Coff; Con; Gels; Ign; Kali-c; Nux-v; Op; Puls). Unable to sleep after 3 pm, having slept well until this time
- Ligament pain / sciatica[2] (Arn; Caust; Ferr; Mag-p; Phyt; Puls; Sep)
- Regulation of milk supply[4] (Calc; Phyt; Puls; Sil)
- Retained placenta, prevention of[5] (Arn)
- Sudden groin pains in pregnancy, with weakness in the legs
- Varicose veins[2,6] (Calc; Carb-v; Ferr; Ham; Lyc; Nux-v; Puls; Sep; Tril; Zinc) especially those of the vulva

Bryonia (Bry) *Bryonia alba.* Other names: White bryony, wild hops, 'the bear'

Prime indications:[7]
- **Much worse from any motion**
- **Stitching, stabbing, pulsating pains**
- **Aggravation from light touch yet amelioration from heavy pressure, e.g. lying on painful part**
- **Chilliness worse in a warm room and better in the open air**
- **Fever with thirst for large quantities of cold water at infrequent intervals**
- **Dryness of mucous and serous membranes**

Additional characteristics:
General
- Does not wish to be moved in any way
- Complaints develop slowly

Emotional
- Wants to be left alone, becoming very irritable when disturbed
- Mental dullness
- Confusion
- Anxious fear of death
- Impetuous
- Delirium
- Sadness
- Hurried

Caused by
- Anger
- Taking cold and getting chilled while perspiring
- Drinking cold drinks when heated
- Becoming warm
- Heat of the sun

Sensations
- Pressure
- Heaviness

Pains
- Bursting
- Burning
- As of a load

Worse
- Morning
- Evening
- Night
- Motion
- Being jolted
- Becoming heated
- Warm room
- After eating
- Stooping

Better
- Pressure
- Lying on painful side
- Cold and warm applications
- Lying down
- Cold drinks

Notes
- Bryonia follows well after Aconite, Ant tart[2] or Nux vomica
- Bryonia is followed well by Kali-carb, Nux vomica, Phosphorus, Pulsatilla or Silica
- If well-indicated Bryonia failed to act, Phytolacca may help

Suggested uses:
- Abdominal pain[6,8] (Acet-ac; Ars; Bell-p; Cimic; Cupr; Puls) due to uterine ligament tension
- Backache[5,6,8,11] (Bell; Calc; Cimic; Ferr; Hyp; Kali-c; Kali-p; Lyc; Merc; Nat-m; Nux-v; Phos; Puls; Sep; Sil; Zinc)
- Excessive lactation[3,6,9] (Bell; Bor; Calc; Cham; Con; Lac-c; Lyc; Phos; Phyt; Ust)
- Eye discharges in infants[8,9] (Acon; Apis; Arg-n; Ars; Bell; Calc; Lyc; Merc; Nat-m; Puls; Zinc)
- Heartburn[11] (Acet-ac; Calc; Carb-v; Caust; Merc; Nat-m; Nux-v; Puls; Zinc)
- Inadequate lactation[2,3,6,8,12] (Acon; Arg-n; Ars; Apis; Bell; Calc; Caust; Dulc; Graph; Ign; Lyc; Phyt; Puls; Sil; Urt-u)
- Mastitis[1,6,7,9,10,12] (Acon; Ars; Apis; Arn; Bell; Calc; Cham; Con; Graph; Lac-c; Lyc; Merc; Phos; Phyt; Puls; Sil). The milk is suppressed or develops too slowly. The breast swells to stony hardness, is reddened, extremely sensitive and heavy. Must support the breast
- Neonatal jaundice[3,6,7,9,11] (Acon; Ars; Cham; Chel; China; Mag-m; Merc; Nux-v; Phos; Sep)
- Phlebitis (Arn; Ham; Puls)
- Postpartum haemorrhage[4,13] (Acet-ac; Acon; Bell; Carb-v; Caul; China; Cinn-m; Ferr; Ham; Ip; Kali-c; Phos; Sab; Sec; Sep; Ust)
- Subinvolution[8] (Arn; Bell; Calc; Carb-v; Caul; Chin; Cimic; Goss; Helon; Op; Puls; Sab; Sec; Sep; Staph; Ust)

Calc carb (Calc) *Calcarea carbonica.* Other names: Middle layer of oyster shell, calcium carbonate, carbonate of lime, $CaCo_3$

Prime indications:[7]
- **Lack of vital heat**
- **Sensation of coldness in single parts**
- **Perspiration of single parts**

- **Aversion to open air**
- **Ailments from effects of strain**

Additional characteristics:

General
- Malaise
- Great relaxation of tissue
- Swollen lymphatic glands
- Craves eggs, indigestible things, raw potatoes, salt
- Profuse perspiration, especially on the head

Emotional
- Mental dullness
- Confusion
- Difficult thinking
- Irritability
- Obstinacy
- Sadness
- Fear of insanity
- Difficulty in verbal expression

Sensations
- Heaviness
- Numbness or heat of single parts

Pains
- Cutting
- Griping
- Stitching
- Pulsating
- Burning

Worse
- Morning
- Waking
- Evening
- Night
- Cold
- Cold air and draughts
- Wet weather
- Bathing
- After eating
- Mental exertion
- Physical exertion

Better
- Warmth
- Lying down
- Lying on painful part

Notes
- Calcarea carbonica follows Belladonna, Chamomilla, China, Conium, Cuprum, Nux vomica or Pulsatilla well
- Calcarea carbonica is followed well by Lycopodium, Nux vomica, Phosphorus or Silica

Suggested uses:
- Anaemia[6] (Alet; Ars; Carb-v; Chin; Cupr; Ferr; Helon; Kali-c; Kali-p; Merc; Nat-m; Phos; Puls; Sep; Staph; Sul-ac; Tril)
- Backache[8,12] (Bell; Bry; Cimic; Ferr; Hyp; Kali-c; Kali-p; Lyc; Merc; Nat-m; Nux-v; Phos; Puls; Sep; Sil; Zinc)
- Candida (Ant-t; Ars; Bor; Nat-m; Merc; Sul-ac)
- Carpal tunnel syndrome (Apis; Ars; Caust; Lyc; Sep)
- Constipation (Caust; Kali-c; Lyc; Nux-v; Op; Sil) in infant[4,8,9,12]
- Cradle cap (Lyc)
- Cramping[3,8,9,12] (Cham; Cupr; Ferr; Ign; Mag-p; Nux-v; Sep; Zinc)
- Excessive lactation[2,6,9] (Bell; Bor; Bry; Cham; Con; Lac-c; Lyc; Phos; Phyt; Ust)
- Eye discharges in infants[8,9,12] (Bry; Lyc; Merc; Nat-m; Puls; Zinc)
- Fear[1,12] (Acon; Arg-n; Ars; Cimic; Gels; Ign; Op; Phos; Puls; Rescue remedy)
- Gestational hypertension (Acet-ac; Apis; Ars; Bell; Ferr; Gels; Helon; Kali-c; Lyc; Merc; Nat-m; Op; Phos; Puls; Sep; Zinc)
- Hair loss after giving birth (Carb-v; Lyc; Nat-m; Sep; Sil)
- Heartburn[2,3,5] (Acet-ac; Bry; Carb-v; Caust; Merc; Nat-m; Nux-v; Puls; Zinc)
- Inadequate lactation[2,6,8,9] (Acon; Arg-n; Ars; Apis; Bell; Bry; Caust; Cham; Dulc; Graph; Ign; Lyc; Phos; Phyt; Puls; Sil; Urt-u)
- Lochia intermittent, returning or prolonged
- Mastitis[1,6,9] (Acon; Ars; Apis; Arn; Bell; Bry; Cham; Con; Graph; Lac-c; Lyc; Merc; Phos; Phyt; Puls; Sil)
- Pruritus vulvae[1,2,3,9,12] (Acon; Ars; Bell; Bor; Coff; Collins; Graph; Ham; Helon; Lyc; Merc; Sep; Sil)
- Regulate milk supply[4] (Bell; Phyt; Puls; Sil)
- Sore, cracked nipples[2,6] (Acet-ac; Arn; Ars; Bell; Cast-eq; Caust; Cham; Graph; Hyp; Lac-c; Lyc; Merc; Phos; Phyt; Puls; Sep; Sil; Staph; Rescue remedy)
- Subinvolution[2,8] (Arn; Bell; Bry; Carb-v; Caul; Chin; Cimic; Goss; Helon; Op; Puls; Sab; Sec; Sep; Staph; Ust)
- Uterine haemorrhage[12] (Acet-ac; Acon; Bell; Bry; Carb-v; Caul; Chin; Ferr; Ham; Cinn-m; Ip; Phos; Sab; Sec; Sep; Ust) of profuse, bright red blood. May occur due to fibroids, after spontaneous abortion or during or after delivery
- Varicose veins[2,6,7,8] (Bell-p; Carb-v; Ferr; Ham; Lyc; Nux-v; Puls; Sep; Tril; Zinc) especially in the thighs, with burning pains and soreness

---

Calendula (Calen) *Calendula officinalis.* Other names: Marigold

---

Prime indications:
- **Torn or ragged wounds**

- Lacerated or suppurating wounds
- Injuries where the skin is broken
- Inflammation and redness with a great deal of discomfort
- Pain is out of proportion to the injury

Additional characteristics:
General
- Sensitive to cold air, particularly in cloudy weather

Sensations
- As if beaten

Worse
- Evening
- Damp weather

Better
- Warmth
- Rest

Note May be alternated with any other remedy that is needed

Suggested uses:
- Episiotomy or tear[3,12] (Acet-ac; Caust; Staph). Calendula tincture can be applied externally to speed the healing process by adding a few drops of tincture to a glass of water. It may sting for a short while! ('Hypercal', a blend of Hypericum and Calendula mother tinctures, is available for the same purpose.)
- After forceps delivery[3] (Arn; Caust; Cham; Hyp; Staph). In this case it is better given internally in potentized form
- Infection of the umbilical cord in an infant who is otherwise healthy[4] (Sil). Best used in aqueous solution and dressed with Calendula ointment afterwards

---

Carbo-veg (Carb-v) *Carbo vegetabilis*, C. Other names: Wood charcoal, carbon

---

Prime indications:[7]
- **Lack of reaction**
- **Mental and physical sluggishness**
- **Weakness and prostration**
- **Icy coldness**
- **Burning pains**
- **Excessive flatulence**
- **Aggravation from extremes of temperature**

Additional characteristics:
General
- Therapeutic range extends from simple ailments to conditions simulating death itself
- Fainting
- Coma
- Cyanosis

- Hardened lymphatic glands, cancers, ulcers
- Offensive discharges

Emotional
- Anxiety
- Indifference
- Weak memory
- Sadness and weeping
- Restlessness

Caused by
- Exhausting acute disease
- Overeating and alcohol
- Late stages of disease

Sensations
- Numbness
- Tingling
- Constriction

Pains
- Pressing
- Tearing
- Stitching

Worse
- Morning
- Evening
- After eating
- Fats, rich food
- Walking in open air
- Clothing around the abdomen
- Hot, humid weather

Better
- Cool air
- Being fanned
- Eructations
- Repose

Note Carbo-veg is followed well by Arsenicum, China, Kali-carb, Lycopodium, Phosphorus, Pulsatilla or Sepia[7]

Suggested uses:
- Anaemia[10,12] (Alet; Ars; Calc; Chin; Cupr; Ferr; Helon; Kali-c; Kali-p; Merc; Nat-m; Phos; Puls; Sep; Staph; Sul-ac; Tril)
- Delayed recovery (Sep) following caesarean section
- Failure to progress[9,13] (Acon; Arn; Bell; Bor; Caul; Cham; Chin; Cimic; Cinn-m; Coff; Cupr; Gels; Ign; Kali-c; Kali-p, Lyc; Mag-m; Nat-m; Nux-v; Op; Puls; Sec; Sep)
- Hair loss after giving birth[2,6] (Calc; Lyc; Nat-m; Sep; Sil)
- Heartburn[12] (Acet-ac; Bry; Calc; Caust; Merc; Nat-m; Nux-v; Puls; Zinc)
- Labour at standstill[9,13] (Acon; Chin; Cimic; Cinn-m; Gels; Nux-v; Op)

- Neonatal respiratory difficulties at delivery[4,13] (Acon; Ant-t; Arn; Ars; Bell; Laur; Op)
- Postpartum haemorrhage[3,4,6,7,10,13] (Acet-ac; Acon; Bell; Bry; Caul; Chin; Cinn-m; Ferr; Ham; Ip; Kali-c; Sab; Sec; Sep; Ust). Aids recovery afterwards[7]
- Subinvolution[8] (Arn; Bell; Bry; Calc; Caul; Chin; Cimic; Goss; Helon; Op; Puls; Sab; Sec; Sep; Staph; Ust)
- Varicose veins[2,6,7,8,9,12,13] (Bell-p; Calc; Ferr; Ham; Lyc; Nux-v; Sep; Tril; Zinc) of leg, thigh and vulva

---

Caulophyllum (Caul) *Caulophyllum thalictroides*. Other names: Blue cohosh, squaw root, papoose root, blueberry root

---

Prime indications:
- **General weakness and exhaustion**
- **Internal trembling**
- **Sharp and intermittent pains**

Additional characteristics:
General
- Rheumatic, experiencing pains in the small joints of the fingers and toes and in the wrists and ankles
- Can scarcely speak from exhaustion

Emotional
- Fretful and easily displeased
- Apprehensive

Caused by
- Exertion

Sensations
- Small joints display stiffness, drawing, aching and swelling on exertion
- Fullness in hypogastric region

Pains
- Cause person to cry out in agony
- Cramp-like
- Uterine contractions shift from place to place, never establishing correctly, thus failing to dilate the cervix or empty the uterus[4]

Worse
- Hot weather
- Lying on back
- Lying on right side

Better
- Pressure
- Bending double
- Lying on left side

Note Where well-indicated Caulophyllum fails to help, Gelsemium may succeed

Suggested uses:
- After pains[2,5,6,9,11,12,13] (Arn; Cham; Cimic; Cupr; Hyp; Kali-c; Mag-p; Nux-v; Puls; Sab; Sec; Sil) across lower abdomen, extending into groins
- Acceleration of labour[4,12,13] (Cimic; Goss; Nat-m; Nux-v)
- Failure to progress[3,4,6,7,9,12,13] (Acon; Arn; Bell; Bor; Carb-v; Cham; Chin; Cimic; Cinn-m; Coff; Cupr; Gels; Ign; Kali-c; Kali-p; Lyc; Mag-m; Nat-m; Nux-v; Op; Puls; Sec; Sep)
- Pain relief during labour (Acon; Arn; Bell; Cham; Cimic; Coff; Cupr; Gels; Ign; Kali-c; Lyc; Mag-m; Mag-p; Nux-v; Puls; Sec; Sep)
- Postpartum haemorrhage[2,4,6,7,8,10,12,13] (Acet-ac; Acon; Bell; Bry; Carb-v; Chin; Cinn-m; Ferr; Ham; Ip; Kali-c; Sab; Sec; Sep; Ust). Passive, with profuse, dark blood
- Prolonged lochia (Calc; Sec)
- Protracted labour due to rigidity of os[4,7]
- Retained placenta[2,8,9,13] (Bell; Cimic; Goss; Ign; Nux-v; Puls; Sab; Sec; Sep)
- Spontaneous abortion[2,6,8,9,11,12,13] (Acon; Alet; Apis; Arn; Bell; Cimic; Ferr; Goss; Helon; Ip; Kali-c; Kali-p; Nux-v; Op; Puls; Sab; Sec; Sep; Tril), due to uterine weakness during first trimester
- Subinvolution[2,8,12] (Arn; Bell; Bry; Calc; Carb-v; Chin; Cimic; Goss; Helon; Op; Puls; Sab; Sec; Sep; Ust)
- Vaginal bleeding during pregnancy (Acon; Arn; Bell; Ign; Op; Puls; Sab; Sec; Sep; Tril)
- Vaginal discharge and candida during pregnancy[2] (Bor; Helon; Nat-m; Merc; Puls; Sep)

Causticum (Caust) *Causticum hahnemanni* (Mostly potassium hydroxide, KOH, prepared from a mixture of calcium hydroxide, Ca(OH)$_2$ and potassium sulphate, K$_2$SO$_4$.) Other names: Potassium hydrate

---

Prime indications:
- **Tendency towards paralysis of any type: paralytic weakness and paralysis of single parts**
- **Great sensitivity to cold**
- **Better in damp weather**
- **Relieves contracted muscles and tendons**

Additional characteristics:
General
- The paralysis may take any form, e.g. facial convulsions or ticks, trembling, twitching, stammering, chorea, etc.
- Anaemic, physically tired, averse to any effort
- Restless at night
- Craves smoked meats, salt and beer and dislikes sweet foods
- May have warts on the tip of the nose or fingertips

Emotionally
- Mentally tired by their anxiety for others
- Very sympathetic, with a great sense of justice
- Introverted and timid
- Pessimistic and forgetful, e.g. 'Did I remember to lock the door before I left the house?'
- Fears dogs and being alone in the dark

Caused by
- Cold and dry winds
- Suppressed grief

Sensations
- Numbness
- Tingling
- Coldness

Pains
- Stitching
- Burning
- Itching
- Tearing

Worse
- Evening
- Night
- Cold
- After eating
- Mental or physical exertion

Better
- Damp weather
- Cold drinks
- Warmth

Notes
- Causticum must not be used before or after Phosphorus
- Causticum is also incompatible with Coffea

Suggested uses:
- Carpal tunnel syndrome[8] (Apis; Ars; Calc; Lyc; Sep)
- Constipation in infant[3,5,6,8,10,11,12] (Calc; Kali-c; Lyc; Nux-v; Op; Sil)
- Constipation in mother[3,5,6,8,10,11,12] (Collins; Cupr; Graph; Ign; Kali-c; Lyc; Mag-m; Mag-p; Nux-v; Op; Phos; Puls; Sab; Sep)
- Episiotomy, after (Acet-ac; Arn; Calen; Staph)
- Frequency of micturition[3,5,6,8] (Ars; Bell; Nat-m; Puls; Sep)
- Heartburn (Acet-ac; Bry; Calc; Carb-v; Merc; Nat-m; Nux-v; Puls; Zinc)
- Inadequate lactation[2,6,8,9] (Acon; Arg-n; Ars; Apis; Bell; Bry; Calc; Cham; Dulc; Graph; Ign; Lyc; Phos; Phyt; Puls; Sil; Urt-u)
- Incontinence[6,8,12] (Arg-n; Arn; Ars; Bell; Tril) especially when walking, coughing, etc.

- Ligament pain/sciatica[3,8,12] (Arn; Bell-p; Ferr; Mag-p; Phyt; Puls; Sep)
- Loss of libido[2,6,8,12] (Graph; Nat-m; Sep)
- Retention of urine, after labour[4,11,12] (Acon; Arn; Ars; Bell; Hyp; Lyc; Op; Sec; Staph) with no desire to micturate
- Sore/cracked nipples[3,4,6,12] (Acet-ac; Acon; Arn; Ars; Bell; Calc; Cast-eq; Cham; Graph; Hyp; Lac-c; Lyc; Merc; Phos; Phyt; Puls; Sep; Sil; Staph; Rescue remedy)

Chamomilla (Cham) *Matricaria chamomilla.* Other names: German chamomile, corn feverfew

---

Prime indications:
- **Touchiness – angry, impossible to please (mental calmness contraindicates this remedy)**
- **Intolerant of slightest pain**
- **Oversensitive**
- **Intense heat**
- **Thirst**
- **Numbness**

Additional characteristics:
General
- Inclined to lie down, but pain and anxiety force her to move about
- Dislikes open air
- Discharges offensive and acrid

Emotional
- Flies into a rage over trivialities and cannot be placated
- Irritated by music, being spoken to, being looked at, the presence of others
- Obstinate
- Impatient
- Discontented
- Capricious
- Sad
- Absent-minded
- Faint

Caused by
- Anger
- Getting chilled in cold, windy weather
- Coffee
- Narcotics
- Dentition

Sensations
- Numbness
- Fullness
- Pressure
- Heat of single parts

Pains
- Tearing
- Cutting
- Pulsating

Worse
- Consolation
- Coffee
- Tobacco
- Sweets
- Emotional excitement
- Mental exertion

Better
- Eating
- Changing position
- Warmth

Notes
- Chamomilla follows Belladonna or Pulsatilla well
- Chamomilla is followed well by Arsenicum, Calcarea carbonica or Pulsatilla

Suggested uses:
- After caesarean (Acet-ac; Arn; Bell-p)
- After pains[2,3,6,7,8,9,11] (Arn; Caul; Cimic; Cupr; Hyp; Kali-c; Mag-p; Nux-v; Puls; Sab; Sec; Sil)
- Colic[3,6,7,9,10,12] (Cupr; Ign; Ip; Mag-m; Mag-p; Nux-v; Sec; Staph)
- Cramping[1,6,8] (Calc; Cupr; Ferr; Ign; Mag-p; Nux-v; Sep; Zinc) in calves[2]
- Excessive lactation[2,9] (Bell; Bor; Bry; Calc; Con; Lac-c; Lyc; Phos; Phyt; Ust)
- Failure to progress[3,6,7,9,12,13] (Acon; Arn; Bell; Bor; Carb-v; Caul; Chin; Cimic; Cinn-m; Coff; Cupr; Gels; Ign; Kali-c; Kali-p; Lyc; Mag-m; Nat-m; Nux-v; Op; Puls; Sec; Sep)
- Hypertension during labour[2] (Acon; Apis; Arn; Bell; Cimic; Gels; Ign; Merc; Nat-m; Op; Puls; Sep)
- Ill-effects of morphine[3,13] or pethidine (Nux-v; Op)
- Inadequate lactation[2,6,7,9] (Acon; Arg-n; Ars; Apis; Bell; Bry; Calc; Caust; Dulc; Graph; Ign; Lyc; Phos; Phyt; Puls; Sil; Urt-u)
- Mastitis[7,9] (Acon; Ars; Apis; Arn; Bell; Bry; Calc; Con; Graph; Lac-c; Merc; Phos; Phyt; Puls; Sil)
- Neonatal jaundice[2,5,6,9] (Acon; Ars; Bry; Chel; Chin; Mag-m; Merc; Nux-v; Phos; Sep)
- Pain relief during labour[3,12] (Acon; Arn; Bell; Caul; Cimic; Coff; Cupr; Gels; Ign; Kali-c; Lyc; Mag-m; Mag-p; Nux-v; Puls; Sec; Sep)
- Sleeplessness in infant[8,9] (Acon; Bell; Phos; Puls)
- Sore, cracked nipples[2,4] (Acet-ac; Acon; Arn; Ars; Bell; Calc; Cast-eq; Caust; Graph; Hyp; Lac-c; Lyc; Merc; Phos; Phyt; Puls; Sep; Sil; Staph; Rescue remedy)

Chelidonium (Chel) *Chelidonium majus.* Other names: Greater celandine

Prime indications:
- **Jaundice of the newborn**
- **Constant pain under inferior angle of right scapula**
- **Great debility and drowsiness after eating and on waking**
- **Sleepiness and yawning**

Additional characteristics:
General
- For liver and venous complaints
- Chilly
- Does not wish to move
- Tired on least exertion
- Yellow face, especially the nose and cheeks
- Skin wilted, sallow, cold and clammy
- Stool may be yellow, pasty, clay-coloured and float in water
- Diarrhoea may alternate with constipation
- One foot may be cold while the other is hot

Emotional
- Strong-minded
- Sceptical

Pains
- Bruised
- Aching

Worse
- Motion
- Touch
- Lying on right side
- 4 am and 4 pm

Better
- After food
- Hot food / drink
- Pressure
- Bending backward

Note Chelidonium is followed well by Lycopodium

Suggested uses:
- Milk diminished[6] (Acon; Arg-n; Ars; Bell; Bry; Calc; Caust; Dulc; Ign; Phyt; Puls; Sil; Urt-u)
- Nausea during pregnancy[6] (Acet-ac; Alet; Ant-t; Ars; Goss; Ip; Nux-v; Phos; Puls; Sep) with desire for food and made better by drinking milk or hot drinks. With sensation of heat in the stomach
- Neonatal jaundice[3,6,10,11,12] (Acon; Ars; Bry; Cham; Chin; Mag-m; Merc; Phos; Sep) where the sclera, face, urine and stool are very yellow, the baby is well in all other respects and there are no symptoms

indicating that another remedy may be more appropriate

China (Chin) *China officinalis* or *Cinchona calisaya*. Other names: Quinine, Peruvian bark, calisaya bark, yellow cinchona, loxa bark, red bark

---

Prime indications:
- **General weakness, debility and oversensitivity**
- **Relaxation of involuntary muscles**
- **Local congestions, general dropsy, oedema**
- **Passive haemorrhage of dark blood**
- **Anaemia with extreme debility**
- **Intermittent fevers**
- **Periodic complaints – on alternate days**

Additional characteristics:
General
- Chilliness
- Lassitude
- Faintness
- Sensitivity to pain, noise and touch
- Rapid, thready pulse
- Tinnitus

Emotional
- Apathy
- Sadness
- Loathing of life
- Abundance of ideas
- Delusions of persecution

Caused by
- Loss of body fluids – haemorrhage, excessive lactation, perspiration, diarrhoea, pus
- Suppressed malaria

Sensations
- Coldness
- Numbness of single parts

Pains
- Tearing
- Pressing
- Stitching

Worse
- Night
- Cold
- Touch
- Open air and draughts
- Cloudy weather
- After eating
- Lying on painful side

Better
- Firm pressure
- After sweating
- Warmth

Notes
- China is followed well by Arsenicum, Calcarea carbonica or Phosphorus
- China follows Belladonna well

Suggested uses:
- Anaemia[5,6,11,13] (Alet; Ars; Calc; Carb-v; Cupr; Ferr; Helon; Kali-c; Kali-p; Merc; Nat-m; Phos; Puls; Sep; Staph; Sul-ac; Tril)
- Depression during pregnancy (Cimic; Con; Ign; Nat-m; Puls; Sep)
- Diarrhoea[3,6,8,9,10] (Ars; Merc; Phos; Puls) during pregnancy
- Failure to progress[6,13] (Acon; Arn; Bell; Bor; Carb-v; Caul; Cham; Cimic; Cinn-m; Coff; Cupr; Gels; Ign; Kali-c; Kali-p; Lyc; Mag-m; Nat-m; Nux-v; Op; Puls; Sec; Sep)
- Labour at standstill[6,13] (Acon; Carb-v; Cimic; Cinn-m; Gels; Nux-v; Op)
- Neonatal jaundice[3,6,8,9,10,11,12] (Acon; Ars; Bry; Cham; Chel; Mag-m; Merc; Nux-v; Phos; Sep)
- Postnatal depression[12] (Cimic; Con; Ign; Nat-m; Puls; Sep)
- Postpartum haemorrhage[3,4,6,8,10,11,12,13] (Acon; Bell; Bry; Carb-v; Caul; Cinn-m; Ferr; Ham; Ip; Phos; Sab; Sec; Sep; Ust) due to atony of the uterus, accompanied by tinnitus, loss of sight, fainting, coldness and blueness of the skin. Intense, throbbing headache and debility follow
- Subinvolution[8] (Arn; Bell; Bry; Calc; Carb-v; Caul; Cimic; Goss; Helon; Op; Puls; Sab; Sec; Sep; Staph; Ust)

Cimicifuga (Cimic) *Cimicifuga racemosa* or *Actaea racemosa*. Other names: Black cohosh, black snake root, bugbane

---

Prime indications:
- **Sighing and deep sadness**
- **Chilly, better in open air**
- **Muscular soreness after exertion causes insomnia**

Additional characteristics:
General
- Trembling
- Nervous shuddering
- Twitching
- Jerking
- Choreic movements

Emotional
- Nervous and hysterical
- As if 'enveloped in a dark cloud'
- Talkative, even during a contraction
- Fear of insanity

Caused by
- Mental strain
- Anxiety
- Fright
- Disappointed love
- Exertion
- Delivery

Sensations
- Bruised
- As though the brain is too large
- As though the top of the head will fly off
- Electric-like shocks
- Numbness

Pains
- Sharp
- Shooting in all directions, e.g. from ovaries upwards, from one ovary to the other or from occiput to vertex

Worse
- Cold
- Draughts
- Excitement

Better
- Warm wraps
- Gentle, continued motion
- Open air
- Eating

Suggested uses:
- Abdominal pain (Acet-ac; Arn; Ars; Bell-p; Bry; Cupr; Puls) due to uterine ligament tension
- Acceleration of labour[4] (Caul; Goss; Nat-m; Nux-v)
- After pains[2,3,7,8] (Arn; Caul; Cham; Cupr; Hyp; Kali-c; Mag-p; Nux-v; Puls; Sab; Sec; Sil) unbearable, centred in the groin
- Backache[3] (Bell; Bry; Calc; Ferr; Hyp; Kali-c; Kali-p; Lyc; Merc; Nat-m; Nux-v; Phos; Puls; Sep; Sil; Zinc)
- Depression during pregnancy[3] (Chin; Con; Ign; Nat-m; Puls; Sep)
- Dizziness and fainting during pregnancy (Ars; Bell; Gels; Ign; Kali-c; Laur; Nat-m; Nux-v; Puls; Sep)
- Failure to progress[7,13] (Acon; Arn; Bell; Bor; Carb-v; Caul; Cham; Chin; Cinn-m; Coff; Cupr; Gels; Ign; Kali-c; Kali-p; Lyc; Mag-m; Nat-m; Nux-v; Op; Puls; Sec; Sep)
- Fear[1,9,13] (Acon; Arg-n; Ars; Caul; Gels; Ign; Op; Phos; Puls; Rescue remedy)

- Hypertension during labour[2] (Acon; Apis; Arn; Bell; Cham; Gels; Ign; Merc; Nat-m; Op; Puls; Sep)
- Labour at standstill[1,13] (Acon; Carb-v; Chin; Cinn-m; Gels; Nux-v; Op)
- Pain relief during labour (Acon; Arn; Bell; Caul; Cham; Coff; Cupr; Gels; Ign; Kali-c; Lyc; Mag-m; Mag-p; Nux-v; Puls; Sec; Sep)
- Retained placenta[2,8] (Bell; Caul; Goss; Ign; Nux-v; Puls; Sab; Sec; Sep)
- Spontaneous abortion[2,7,8,13] in 12th week (Acon; Alet; Apis; Arn; Bell; Caul; Ferr; Goss; Helon; Ip; Kali-c; Kali-p; Nux-v; Op; Puls; Sab; Sec; Sep; Tril). Pains shoot from one side of the pelvis to the other. Accompanied by fainting and shivering
- Subinvolution[2,8] (Arn; Bell; Bry; Calc; Carb-v; Caul; Chin; Goss; Helon; Op; Puls; Sab; Sec; Sep; Staph; Ust) may occur after spontaneous abortion
- Postnatal depression[2,3,8] (Chin; Con; Ign; Nat-m; Puls; Sep) where she feels imprisoned by having baby to take care of
- Puerperal mania[2] (Ars; Bell; Cupr; Lyc; Sec; Zinc)

Cinnamomum (Cinn-m) *Cinnamomum majus*. Other name: Cinnamon

Prime indications:
- **Profuse, bright red haemorrhage**
- **Repeated small haemorrhages during gestation and puerperal state**
- **Metrorrhagia**

Additional characteristics:
General
- Always worse from lifting or exertion

Emotional
- Prone to hysteria

Caused by
- False step
- Strain
- Lifting
- Overstretching arms

Worse
- Talking, which may bring on hysterical attack
- Afternoon
- Evening up until midnight

Suggested uses:
- Failure to progress during labour[9,13] (Acon; Arn; Bell; Bor; Carb-v; Caul; Cham; China; Cimic; Coff; Cupr; Gels; Ign; Kali-c; Kali-p; Lyc; Mag-m; Nat-m; Nux-v; Op; Puls; Sec; Sep). Contractions are ineffectual, weak or ceasing

- Labour at standstill[9,13] (Acon; Carb-v; China; Cimic; Gels; Nux-v; Op)
- Postpartum haemorrhage[2,4,6,8,13] (Acet-ac; Acon; Bell; Bry; Carb-v; Caul; China; Ferr; Ham; Ip; Kali-c; Phos; Sab; Sec; Sep; Ust)
- Secondary postpartum haemorrhage[9,13] (Kali-c; Sab; Ust) without excessive flow of blood
- Severe flooding in primipara after first few pains

Coffea (Coff) *Coffea cruda* or *Coffea arabica*. Other names: Raw coffee bean, mocha bean

Prime indications:
- **Hypersensitive**
- **All senses are more acute – sight, hearing, smell, taste and touch**
- **Cannot bear pain**

Additional characteristics:
General
- Head red and hot, with shiny cheeks
- Pupils dilated

Emotional
- Euphoric, yet despairing with pain
- May howl, cry and toss about with pain
- Tearful
- Moaning
- Fearful of painful death
- Fainting from fright
- Infants cannot bear to be carried about

Caused by
- Excitement
- Joy

Sensations
- As if brain were bruised

Worse
- Draughts
- Open air
- Touch

Better
- Warmth
- Cold water
- Lying down

Suggested uses:
- Failure to progress during labour[9,13] (Acon; Arn; Bell; Bor; Carb-v; Caul; Cham; Chin; Cupr; Gels; Ign; Kali-c; Kali-p; Lyc; Mag-m; Nat-m; Nux-v; Op; Puls; Sec; Sep) with talkativeness, constant complaining and fear of death. Contractions felt only in the back, irregular, severe, stopping or slowing down

- Insomnia[2,3,4,5,6,8,9,12] (Acon; Bell; Bell-p; Con; Gels; Ign; Kali-c; Nux-v; Op; Puls) during pregnancy and/or after delivery, from good news
- Pain relief during labour (Acon; Arn; Bell; Caul; Cham; Cimic; Cupr; Gels; Ign; Kali-c; Lyc; Mag-m; Mag-p; Nux-v; Puls; Sec; Sep)
- Pruritus vulvae[2,6,12] (Acon; Ars; Bell; Bor; Calc; Collins; Graph; Ham; Helon; Lyc; Merc; Sep; Sil), too sensitive to scratch

Gelsemium (Gels) *Gelsemium sempervirens*. Other names: Yellow jasmine

Prime indications:[7]
- **Mental and physical relaxation, weakness and slowness**
- **Paralysis accompanied by numbness, tingling and coldness of affected part**
- **Drowsiness and absence of thirst during fever**
- **Cold extremities and hot head**
- **Involuntary stools from fright or anticipating an ordeal**
- **Complaints accompanied by red face, drooping eye lids, dilated pupils and profuse urination**
- **Trembling**

Additional characteristics:
General
- Tired and weary, wants to lie down

Emotional
- Hysterical
- Irritable, sensitive and excitable
- Timid
- Sad, indifferent
- Fears death, the future, being alone and losing control

Caused by
- Fright
- Shock
- Grief

Sensations
- Heaviness
- Fullness
- Enlargement of the head

Pains
- Sharp
- Stitching
- Pressing
- Aching
- Heavy
- Bruised soreness

Worse
- Emotional excitement
- During thunderstorm
- Morning
- Warm, wet weather
- Motion

Better
- Sweating
- Alcohol
- Micturition

Note Gelsemium often succeeds where well-indicated Caulophyllum has not helped

Suggested uses:
- Dizziness and fainting during pregnancy[5,6,8,12] (Ars; Bell; Cimic; Ign; Kali-c; Laur; Nat-m; Nux-v; Puls; Sep)
- Failure to progress[3,6,9,12,13] (Acon; Arn; Bell; Bor; Carb-v; Caul; Cham; Chin; Cimic; Coff; Cupr; Ign; Kali-c; Kali-p; Lyc; Mag-m; Nat-m; Nux-v; Op; Puls; Sec; Sep). Os spasmodically contracted and feels like a hard, unyielding ring. Pains weak or absent. Face flushes with every pain
- Fear[1,3,6,11,12] (Acon; Arg-n; Ars; Calc; Cimic; Con; Op; Phos; Puls; Rescue remedy)
- Gestational hypertension (Acet-ac; Apis; Ars; Bell; Calc; Ferr; Helon; Kali-c; Lyc; Merc; Nat-m; Op; Phos; Puls; Sep; Zinc)
- Hypertension during labour[2] (Acon; Apis; Arn; Bell; Cham; Cimic; Ign; Merc; Nat-m; Op; Puls; Sep)
- Insomnia[3,4,5,9,12,13] (Acon; Bell; Bell-p; Coff; Con; Ign; Kali-c; Nux-v; Op; Puls)
- Labour at standstill[3,7,9] (Acon; Carb-v; Chin; Cimic; Cinn-m; Nux-v; Op). Complete atony of uterus during labour with cervix as soft as putty. Woman exhausted, stupid and drowsy even though in labour for a short time
- Pain relief during labour[12] (Acon; Arn; Bell; Caul; Cham; Cimic; Coff; Cupr; Ign; Kali-c; Lyc; Mag-m; Mag-p; Nux-v; Puls; Sec; Sep)
- Proteinuria[2,4,6,7,8,9] (Apis; Ars; Bell; Ferr; Helon; Kali-c; Lyc; Merc; Nat-m; Phos; Sab; Sep)

Graphites (Graph). Other names: plumbago, black lead

Prime indications:
- **Paralytic weakness and relaxation of tissues**
- **Acrid discharges**
- **Cracks and fissures of the skin especially in the folds of skin around the joints and orifices, i.e. corners of the mouth, finger tips, between the toes, bends of the joints, behind the ears, nails**
- **Skin problems of some sort**

Additional characteristics:
General
- Chilly
- Constipated
- Lazy
- Obese
- Skin eruptions may be eczematous, moist and crusty or itching and discharging sticky fluid
- Even if there are no eruptions, the skin is rough, dry and poorly nourished
- Nails thickened and deformed, may be black

Emotional
- Weeping
- Timidity
- Sadness
- Apprehension

Worse
- Night
- Cold
- Warm room
- Warmth of bed
- Cold draught
- Open air
- Music

Better
- Warmth
- After eating

Notes
- Graphites follows well after Calcarea carbonica, Lycopodium, Pulsatilla or Sepia
- Graphites is followed well by Lycopodium and Silica

Suggested uses:
- Constipation[3,5,6,9,10,11,12] (Caust; Collins; Cupr; Ign; Kali-c; Lyc; Mag-m; Mag-p; Nux-v; Op; Phos; Puls; Sab; Sep). Stool and urine have a sour odour
- Inadequate lactation (Acon; Apis; Arg-n; Ars; Bell; Bry; Calc; Caust; Dulc; Ign; Lyc; Phyt; Puls; Sil; Urt-u)
- Loss of libido[2,3,6,8,12] (Caust; Nat-m; Sep)
- Mastitis[6] (Acon; Apis; Arn; Ars; Bell; Bry; Calc; Cham; Con; Lac-c; Lyc; Merc; Phos; Phyt; Puls; Sil)
- Pruritus vulvae[2,6,9] (Acon; Ars; Bor; Calc; Coff; Collins; Ham; Helon; Lyc; Merc; Sep; Sil)
- Slow recovery following labour[9]
- Sore nipples (Acet-ac; Acon; Arn; Ars; Bell; Calc; Cast-eq; Caust; Cham; Hyp; Lac-c; Lyc; Merc; Phos; Phyt; Puls; Sep; Sil; Staph; Rescue remedy) with deep cracks

---

Ipecac (Ip) *Cephaelis ipecacuanha.* **Other name: Ipecac root**

Prime indications:[7]
- **Persistent nausea**

- **Nausea with all complaints**
- **Clean or thinly coated tongue**
- **Thirstlessness**
- **Profuse secretion of mucus in larynx, trachea and bronchi**
- **Copious arterial haemorrhage**

Additional characteristics:
General
- History of haemorrhage

Emotional
- Wants something, but knows not what
- Sulks
- Irritable
- Easily offended

Caused by
- Eating rich, indigestible foods
- Eating pork, pastry, ice-cream or sweets
- After anger or humiliation

Pains
- Cutting
- Crushing
- Griping

Worse
- Night
- Warmth
- Cold
- Dampness
- Motion
- After eating

Better
- Open air
- Rest
- Cold drinks

Notes
- Ipecac is followed well by Arsenicum, Belladonna, Bryonia, Calcarea carbonica, Chamomilla, China, Cuprum, Ignatia, Nux vomica, Phosphorus, Pulsatilla or Sepia
- Ipecac follows Arnica well

Suggested uses:
- Colic (Cham; Cupr; Ign; Mag-m; Mag-p; Nux-v; Sec; Staph)
- Nausea[2,3,4,5,8,9,12,13] (Acet-ac; Alet; Ant-t; Ars; Chel; Goss; Nux-v; Phos; Puls; Sep) accompanied by weakness, disgust for cold food, cold perspiration especially on the face and profuse salivation. Not relieved by vomiting
- Bleeding during pregnancy[13] (Alet; Apis; Caul; Cimic; Ferr; Goss; Helon; Kali-c; Nux-v; Sab; Sec; Sep; Tril)

with sharp pain in umbilical region, running down into the uterus, with nausea and faintness
- Postpartum haemorrhage[2,3,4,5,6,7,8,10,11,12,13] (Acet-ac; Acon; Bell; Bry; Carb-v; Caul; Chin; Cinn-m; Ferr; Ham; Kali-c; Phos; Sab; Sec; Sep; Ust) accompanied by nausea, faintness and cold sweat, oppression of the chest, gasping, pallor, whiteness of the lips and even the tongue. The blood coagulates quickly
- Spontaneous abortion[2,3,7,8,9,12,13] (Acon; Alet; Apis; Arn; Bell; Caul; Cimic; Ferr; Goss; Helon; Kali-c; Kali-p; Nux-v; Op; Puls; Sab; Sec; Sep; Tril) in 6th week[9]

Kali carb (Kali-c) *Potassium carbonicum*. Other names: Potash, potassium carbonate K_2CO_3, pearl ash, salt of tartar

---

and

Kali phos (Kali-p) *Potassium phosphoricum*. Other names: Phosphate of potash, potassium phosphate

---

These are two of the potash salts, which share common characteristics, including:

- **congestion, inflammation and ulceration of mucous membranes**
- **oedematous swellings**
- **increased and altered mucous discharges**
- **papular and pustular eruptions**
- **worse after midnight**
- **chilly**
- **sensitive to cold air.**

Additional shared characteristics:
General
- Lassitude and weakness
- Heaviness of the extremities
- Twitching, jerking, choreic movements and convulsions

Emotional
- Timid and apprehensive – startled easily by noise or touch
- Conservative, down to earth with strong moral sense

Caused by
- Mental and physical exertion
- Sexual intercouse

Pains
- Stitching
- Shooting

Worse
- Motion

Better
- Warmth
- Warm applications

Kali carb (Kali-c)

Prime characteristics (in addition to those mentioned above):
General
- Dryness and burning
- Marked sensitivity to cold air
- Oedema of lower extremities or of one foot only
- Bag-like swelling above the upper eyelids

Emotional
- Dogmatic, with fear of losing control

Pains
- Darting
- Cutting

Worse
- 3 am
- 3–5 am
- Cold draughts
- Open air
- After eating
- Lying on painful side

Better
- From eructations
- Sitting bent

Note Kali carb follows Bryonia or Phosphorus well

Suggested uses:
- After pains[2,8,9] (Arn; Caul; Cham; Cimic; Cupr; Hyp; Mag-p; Nux-v; Puls; Sab; Sec; Sil)
- Anaemia[6,10,12] (Alet; Ars; Calc; Carb-v; Chin; Cupr; Ferr; Helon; Kali-p; Merc; Nat-m; Phos; Puls; Sep; Staph; Sul-ac; Tril)
- Backache[2,3,5,6,8,10,11,12,13] (Bell; Bry; Calc; Cimic; Ferr; Hyp; Kali-p; Lyc; Merc; Nat-m; Phos; Puls; Sep; Sil; Zinc). Must lie down for immediate relief
- Constipation[3,8,9,11,12] (Caust; Collins; Cupr; Graph; Ign; Lyc; Mag-m; Mag-p; Nux-v; Op; Phos; Puls; Sab; Sep)
- Constipation in infant[8,9,11,12] (Calc; Caust; Lyc; Nux-v; Op; Sil)
- Dizziness and fainting[9,12] (Ars; Bell; Cimic; Gels; Ign; Laur; Nat-m; Nux-v; Puls; Sep)
- Failure to progress[3,6,9,12,13] (Acon; Arn; Bell; Bor; Carb-v; Caul; Cham; Chin; Cimic; Cinn-m; Coff; Cupr; Gels; Ign; Kali-p; Lyc; Mag-m; Nat-m; Nux-v; Op; Puls; Sec; Sep)
- Gestational hypertension[3,12] (Acet-ac; Apis; Ars; Bell; Calc; Ferr; Gels; Helon; Lyc; Merc; Nat-m; Op; Phos; Puls; Sep; Zinc)
- Haemorrhoids[1,3,6,9] (Ars; Collins; Ham; Hyp; Ign; Lyc; Nat-m; Nux-v; Puls; Sab; Sep; Staph), especially postpartum
- Insomnia (Acon; Bell; Bell-p; Coff; Gels; Ign; Nux-v; Op; Puls), especially in the latter part of pregnancy
- Pain relief during labour[12] (Acon; Arn; Bell; Caul; Cham; Cimic; Coff; Cupr; Gels; Ign; Lyc; Mag-m; Mag-p; Nux-v; Puls; Sec; Sep)
- Postpartum haemorrhage[2,6,8,13] (Acon; Bell; Bry; Carb-v; Caul; Chin; Cinn-m; Ferr; Ham; Phos; Sab; Sec; Sep; Ust)
- Proteinuria[3,8,9] (Apis; Ars; Bell; Ferr; Gels; Helon; Lyc; Merc; Nat-m; Phos; Sab; Sep)
- Secondary postpartum haemorrhage[6,9,13] (Cinn-m; Sab; Ust)
- Spontaneous abortion[2,3,6,8,9] (Acon; Alet; Apis; Arn; Bell; Caul; Cimic; Ferr; Goss; Helon; Ip; Kali-p; Nux-v; Op; Sab; Sec; Sep; Tril) at 8–12 weeks

---

Kali phos (Kali-p)

Prime indications (in addition to those mentioned above):
General
- Nervous exhaustion (neurasthenia)

Emotional
- Nervous dread
- Lethargy
- Wants to be alone
- Irritable and tearful
- May be unable to recall words or people's names
- May be cruel to her husband or baby

Worse
- Worry
- Cold draughts

Better
- Eating

Pains
- Stitching
- Burning
- Tearing
- Followed by exhaustion

Suggested uses:
- Anaemia[6] (Alet; Ars; Calc; Carb-v; Chin; Cupr; Ferr; Helon; Kali-c; Merc; Nat-m; Phos; Puls; Sep; Staph; Sul-ac; Tril)
- Backache[8] (Bell; Bry; Calc; Cimic; Ferr; Hyp; Kali-c; Lyc; Merc; Nat-m; Nux-v; Phos; Puls; Sep; Sil; Zinc)
- Failure to progress[3,13] (Acon; Arn; Bell; Bor; Carb-v;

Caul; Cham; Chin; Cimic; Cinn-m; Coff; Cupr; Gels; Ign; Kali-c; Lyc; Mag-m; Nat-m; Nux-v; Op; Puls; Sec; Sep)
- Spontaneous abortion[8] (Acon; Alet; Apis; Arn; Bell; Caul; Cimic; Ferr; Goss; Helon; Ip; Kali-c; Nux-v; Op; Sab; Sec; Sep; Tril)
- Vaginal bleeding during pregnancy (Acon; Arn; Bell; Caul; Ign; Kali-c; Op; Puls; Sab; Sec; Sep; Tril)

Lycopodium (Lyc) *Lycopodium clavatum*. Other names: Club moss, wolf's claw, stag horn, witch meal

---

Prime indications:[7]
- **Mental and physical weakness**
- **Complaints occur on the right side of the body**
- **Complaints appear on the right side of the body and then extend to the left**
- **Excessive flatulence**
- **Worse from 4–8 pm**
- **Red sand in the urine**
- **Fan-like motion of the ali nasi**
- **Hunger with sudden satiety**

Additional characteristics:
General
- Feeble physique
- Predisposition to pulmonary and hepatic problems

Emotional
- Irritable
- Malicious
- Seeks a quarrel
- Intolerant of contradiction
- Restless
- Anxious and fearful yet haughty and domineering at times
- Timid
- Suspicious
- Dislikes company, yet is afraid to be alone, therefore is anxious to have someone in the next room or at ready call
- Confused
- Unable to concentrate or remember the meaning of words

Caused by
- Anger
- Fright
- Mental exertion
- Overeating
- Grande multiparity

Sensations
- Numbness/numbness of single parts
- Internal tension

- Dryness of mucous membranes
- Pulsation

Pains
- Tearing
- Cutting
- Burning
- Pressing

Worse
- Mental exertion
- Cold air
- Cold drinks
- Warmth

Better
- Open air
- Uncovering
- Warm drinks
- Motion
- Eructations
- Lying on left side

Notes
- Lycopodium is followed well by Graphites, Phosphorus, Silica or Pulsatilla
- Lycopodium follows well after Calcarea carbonica, Carbo veg, Chelidonium, Graphites or Nux vomica

Suggested uses:
- Backache[3,7,8,11,12] (Bell; Bry; Calc; Cimic; Ferr; Hyp; Kali-c; Kali-p; Merc; Nat-m; Nux-v; Phos; Puls; Sep; Sil; Zinc)
- Carpal tunnel syndrome[3,8,12] (Apis; Ars; Calc; Caust; Sep)
- Constipation[2,3,6,7,8,9,11,12] during pregnancy[5] (Caust; Collins; Cupr; Graph; Ign; Kali-c; Mag-m; Mag-p; Nux-v; Op; Phos; Puls; Sab; Sep) and also in infants.[9] (Calc; Caust; Kali-c; Nux-v; Op; Sil)
- Cracked nipples (Cast-eq; Caust; Cham; Graph; Lac-c; Phyt; Sep; Sil)
- Cradle cap with moist, scaly eruptions behind the ears and in the folds of the skin (Calc)
- Eye discharges in infant[8,9] (Acon; Apis; Ars; Bell; Bry; Calc; Nat-m; Puls; Zinc)
- Failure to progress[13] (Acon; Arn; Bell; Bor; Carb-v; Caul; Cham; Chin; Cimic; Cinn-m; Coff; Cupr; Gels; Ign; Kali-c; Kali-p; Mag-m; Nat-m; Nux-v; Op; Puls; Sec; Sep)
- Gestational hypertension[3,12] (Acet-ac; Apis; Ars; Bell; Calc; Ferr; Gels; Helon; Kali-c; Merc; Nat-m; Op; Phos; Puls; Sep; Zinc)
- Haemorrhoids[2,6,7,8,9,12] (Ars; Collins; Ham; Hyp; Ign; Kali-c; Nat-m; Nux-v; Puls; Sab; Sep; Staph) which protrude and bleed easily even if there is no

constipation. The anus is sore and surrounded by a moist, itching eruption
- Hair loss after giving birth[8] (Calc; Carb-v; Nat-m; Sep; Sil)
- Inadequate lactation (Acon; Apis; Arg-n; Ars; Bell; Bry; Calc; Caust; Cham; Dulc; Graph; Ign; Phos; Phyt; Puls; Sil; Urt-u)
- Mastitis[6] (Acon; Apis; Arn; Ars; Bell; Bry; Cham; Con; Graph; Lac-c; Merc; Phos; Phyt; Puls; Sil)
- Pain relief during labour (Acon; Arn; Bell; Caul; Cham; Cimic; Coff; Cupr; Gels; Ign; Kali-c; Mag-m; Mag-p; Nux-v; Puls; Sec; Sep)
- Precipitate labour[9]
- Proteinuria[4,6,8,9] (Apis; Ars; Bell; Ferr; Gels; Helon; Kali-c; Merc; Nat-m; Phos; Sab; Sep)
- Pruritus vulvae[6,9] (Acon; Ars; Bell; Bor; Calc; Coff; Collins; Graph; Ham; Helon; Merc; Sep; Sil)
- Puerperal mania[7] (Ars; Bell; Cimic; Cupr; Sec; Zinc) characterized by a superiority complex. May exhibit unreasonable fear of the opposite sex or have sexual desire mounting to nymphomania. Hysterical, laughs and cries alternately, starts at every little noise and is in despair
- Retention of urine[3,13] (Acon; Arn; Ars; Bell; Caust; Op; Sec; Staph)
- Sore, cracked nipples[1,4,9,12] (Acet-ac; Acon; Arn; Ars; Bell; Calc; Cast-eq; Caust; Cham; Graph; Hyp; Merc; Phos; Phyt; Puls; Sep; Sil; Staph; Rescue remedy)
- Varicose veins[2,6,8,9,12] (Bell-p; Calc; Carb-v; Ferr; Ham; Nux-v; Sep; Tril; Zinc) of leg, thigh and vulva

---

Nat mur (Nat-m) *Natrum muriaticum.* Other names: Common salt, sodium chloride, NaCl

---

Prime indications:
- **Constant dwelling on past unpleasant occurrences**
- **Irritability, depression and restlessness combined and made worse from consolation**
- **Emaciation while eating well**
- **Herpetic eruptions**
- **Craves salt and savouries, but worse from fats or bread**
- **Periodicity**
- **Worse between 10 and 11 am**

Additional characteristics:
General
- Chilly
- Liable to take cold easily
- States of weakness are accompanied by mental and nervous sensitivity and a deep sadness
- Weakness, trembling and fainting
- Jerking of body from palpitations, chorea or convulsions
- Profuse perspiration and mucous discharges

Emotional
- Mood may alternate, with the sadness, anxiety and fear suddenly giving way to silly and inappropriate laughter
- Weeping
- Despair
- Wants to be alone
- Indifferent
- Lazy
- Angered easily
- Offended easily
- Startled easily
- Hurried manner
- Hysteria
- Confusion
- Dullness
- Mistakes in speaking
- Anxious about the future; about robbers or burglars

Caused by
- Any distressing emotion, e.g. grief, embarrassment, anger, fright
- Heat of the sun

Sensations
- Heat
- Heaviness
- Numbness of parts

Pains
- Pulsating
- Tearing
- Stitching
- Jerking
- Pressing
- Burning

Worse
- Consolation
- Conversation
- Mental or physical exertion
- Heat of the sun
- Morning 10–11 am

Better
- Perspiration
- Lying down
- Fasting

Note Natrum muriaticum is followed well by Sepia

Suggested uses:
- Acceleration of labour[13] (Caul; Cimic; Goss; Nux-v)
- Anaemia[5,6,7,10,11] (Alet; Ars; Calc; Carb-v; Chin; Cupr; Ferr; Helon; Kali-c; Kali-p; Merc; Phos; Puls; Sep; Staph; Sul-ac; Tril)
- Backache[3,7,8,11,12] (Bell; Bry; Calc; Cimic; Ferr; Hyp;

Kali-c; Kali-p; Lyc; Merc; Nux-v; Phos; Puls; Sep; Sil; Zinc)
- Candida[6,8] (Ant-t; Ars; Bor; Calc; Helon; Merc; Puls; Sep; Sul-ac), especially on the tongue and gums
- Dizziness and fainting[5,6,8] (Ars; Bell; Cimic; Gels; Ign; Kali-c; Laur; Nux-v; Puls; Sep)
- Eye discharges in infants[6,8] (Acon; Apis; Arg-n; Ars; Bell; Bry; Calc; Lyc; Puls; Zinc)
- Failure to progress[6,9,13] (Acon; Arn; Bell; Bor; Carb-v; Caul; Cham; Chin; Cimic; Cinn-m; Coff; Cupr; Gels; Ign; Kali-c; Kali-p; Lyc; Mag-m; Nux-v; Op; Puls; Sec; Sep)
- Frequency of micturition[8,13] (Ars; Bell; Caust; Puls; Sep)
- Gestational hypertension (Acet-ac; Apis; Ars; Bell; Calc; Ferr; Gels; Helon; Kali-c; Lyc; Merc; Op; Phos; Puls; Sep; Zinc)
- Haemorrhoids[1,6,8,9] (Ars; Collins; Ham; Hyp; Ign; Kali-c; Lyc; Nux-v; Puls; Sab; Sep; Staph)
- Hair loss after giving birth[2,6] (Calc; Carb-v; Lyc; Sep; Sil), during lactation[6,9]
- Heartburn[7,8,9,12] (Acet-ac; Bry; Calc; Carb-v; Caust; Merc; Nux-v; Puls; Zinc)
- Hypertension during pregnancy (Acon; Apis; Arn; Bell; Cham; Cimic; Gels; Ign; Merc; Op; Puls; Sep)
- Loss of libido[1,2,3,6,8,12] (Caust; Graph; Sep)
- Postpartum depression[2,6,7,8] (Chin; Cimic; Con; Ign; Puls; Sep)
- Proteinuria[6,8,9] (Apis; Ars; Bell; Gels; Kali-c; Lyc; Phos; Sep)

Nux vomica (Nux-v) *Strychnos nux vomica*. Other names: Poison nut, Quaker buttons

Prime indications:
- **Hypersensitivity of all the senses, especially to noise, strong light, odours and pain**
- **Marked irritability**
- **Frequent ineffectual urging (stool, micturition and work)**
- **Craving for stimulants**
- **Worse in the early morning**

Additional characteristics:
General
- Chilly
- Suffering from mental strain
- Usually employed in sedentary occupation
- Tendency to indulge in rich spicy food and alcohol
- Lassitude
- Spasms and jerking of muscles

Emotional
- Music or singing make the person angry
- Abnormal reflexes (increased)
- Impatient
- Malicious
- Impetuous
- Intolerant of contradiction
- Morose
- Rude
- Suspicious
- Dislikes company
- Concentration difficult
- Confusion
- Mania
- Hysteria

Caused by
- Anger
- Excessive mental labour
- Loss of sleep
- 'Overindulgence'

Sensations
- Heaviness
- Internal tension
- As if ants were crawling

Pains
- Bruised soreness
- Sharp
- Biting
- Jerking
- Paralytic
- Pressing

Worse
- Touch or tight clothing
- After midnight
- Cold and cold air
- Uncovering
- After eating
- Cold food
- Motion or being jolted

Better
- Warmth
- Warm drinks
- Wet weather
- Lying down

Notes
- Nux vomica is followed well by Bryonia, Lycopodium or Pulsatilla
- Nux vomica follows well after Arsenicum, Bryonia,[7] Calcarea carbonica,[7] Ipecac, Phosphorus or Sepia
- Nux vomica goes well either before or after Zinc
- Ignatia should not be used before or after Nux vomica

Suggested uses:
- Abdominal pain[8] (Acet-ac; Arn; Ars; Cupr; Puls; Sep; Staph) due to fetal movements

- Acceleration of labour[13] (Caul; Cimic; Goss; Nat-m)
- After pains[2,6,8,9,11,13] (Arn; Caul; Cham; Cimic; Cupr; Hyp; Mag-p; Puls; Sab; Sec; Sil)
- Backache[3,5,6,8,10,12] (Bell; Bry; Calc; Cimic; Ferr; Hyp; Kali-c; Kali-p; Lyc; Merc; Nat-m; Phos; Puls; Sep; Sil; Zinc)
- Colic[6,9,12] (Cham; Cupr; Ign; Ip; Mag-m; Mag-p; Sec; Staph)
- Constipation[2,3,4,5,6,7,8,9,10,11,12] during pregnancy (Caust; Collins; Cupr; Graph; Ign; Kali-c; Lyc; Mag-m; Mag-p; Op; Phos; Puls; Sab; Sep). Also in infants[9] (Calc; Caust; Kali-c; Lyc; Op; Sil)
- Cramping[1,2,3,5,6,8,11] (Calc; Cham; Cupr; Ferr; Ign; Mag-p; Sep; Zinc)
- Dizziness and fainting during pregnancy[2,6,8,10,12] (Ars; Bell; Cimic; Gels; Ign; Kali-c; Laur; Puls; Sep)
- Failure to progress[6,9,12,13] (Acon; Arn; Bell; Bor; Carb-v; Caul; Cham; Chin; Cimic; Cinn-m; Coff; Cupr; Gels; Ign; Kali-c; Kali-p; Lyc; Mag-m; Nat-m; Op; Puls; Sec; Sep)
- Haemorrhoids[1,2,3,6,7,8,9,10,11,12] (Ars; Collins; Ham; Ign; Kali-c; Lyc; Nat-m; Puls; Sab; Sep; Staph), especially postpartum
- Heartburn[2,3,11,12] (Acet-ac; Bry; Calc; Carb-v; Caust; Merc; Nat-m; Puls; Zinc)
- Ill-effects of drugs administered during and after labour[3,12] (Acet-ac; Cham; Op; Phos; Sec); where a general detox is required
- Induction of labour (Caul; Cimic; Goss; Nat-m)
- Insomnia[2,3,4,9] (Acon; Bell; Bell-p; Coff; Con; Gels; Ign; Kali-c; Op; Puls) from mental strain
- Labour at standstill[9] (Acon; Carb-v; Chin; Cimic; Gels; Op)
- Nausea and vomiting[2,3,5,8,11,12] (Acet-ac; Alet; Ant-t; Chel; Goss; Ip; Phos; Puls; Sep), gagging and vomiting every morning after the simplest foods
- Neonatal jaundice[3,7,9] (Acon; Ars; Bry; Cham; Chel; Chin; Mag-m; Merc; Phos; Sep)
- Pain relief during labour[12] (Acon; Arn; Bell; Caul; Cham; Cimic; Coff; Cupr; Gels; Ign; Kali-c; Lyc; Mag-m; Mag-p; Puls; Sec; Sep)
- Retained placenta[8] (Bell; Caul; Cimic; Goss; Puls; Sab; Sec; Sep) where extreme pains impede expulsion
- Spontaneous abortion[2,3,8,9,12] (Acon; Alet; Apis; Arn; Bell; Caul; Cimic; Ferr; Goss; Helon; Kali-c; Kali-p; Op; Puls; Sab; Sec; Sep; Tril) between 12–16 weeks
- Varicose veins of leg and vulva[8,9] (Bell-p; Calc; Carb-v; Ferr; Ham; Lyc; Sep; Tril; Zinc).

Opium (Op) *Papaver somniferum*. Other names: Opium poppy, white poppy, maw seed

---

Prime indications:
- **Abnormal absence of pain – secretion, reaction, moral sense, judgement**

- **Fear, fright and shock that remain**
- **Wants nothing, can do without food or drink**

Additional characteristics:
General
- Sensitive hearing, e.g. at night can 'hear a clock 10 miles away'
- Drowsy, apathetic, confused, in a stupor
- Face bloated, dark red with distorted features
- Pupils contracted
- Hot, with hot perspiration[4]

Emotional
- Uncontrolled imagination and anxiety neurosis, e.g. may hire someone to watch the house
- Rash, bold and fearless

Worse
- Motion
- Stimulus
- Warmth
- While perspiring
- From fear
- Night

Better
- During sleep
- After sleep
- Cold
- Constant walking
- Open air

Suggested uses:
- Constipation during pregnancy[2,4,5,6,8,9,11,12] (Calc; Caust; Collins; Cupr; Graph; Ign; Kali-c; Lyc; Mag-m; Mag-p; Nux-v; Phos; Puls; Sab; Sep) with no desire for stool. Also in infants[9] (Calc; Caust; Kali-c; Lyc; Nux-v; Sil)
- Failure to progress during labour[3,6,9] (Acon; Arn; Bell; Carb-v; Caul; Cham; Chin; Cimic; Cinn-m; Coff; Gels; Kali-c; Kali-p; Lyc; Nat-m; Nux-v; Puls; Sec; Sep)
- Fear[1,3,4] (Acon; Arg-n; Ars; Calc; Gels; Ign; Phos; Puls; Rescue remedy)
- Gestational hypertension[3] (Acet-ac; Apis; Ars; Bell; Calc; Ferr; Gels; Helon; Kali-c; Lyc; Merc; Nat-m; Phos; Puls; Sep; Zinc)
- Hypertension during labour[2] (Acon; Apis; Arn; Bell; Cham; Cimic; Gels; Ign; Merc; Nat-m; Puls; Sep)
- Ill-effects of morphine, pethidine and general anaesthetic (Acet-ac; Cham; Nux-v; Phos; Sec)
- Insomnia[3,4,6,8,12] (Acon; Bell; Bell-p; Coff; Con; Gels; Ign; Kali-c; Nux-v; Puls) with acute hearing and excessive wakefulness
- Labour at standstill[3,6,9,12] (Acon; Carb-v; Chin; Cimic; Cinn-m; Gels; Nux-v)
- Neonatal respiratory difficulties at delivery[8,13] (Acon; Ant-t; Arn; Ars; Bell; Carb-v; Laur)

- Recovering from caesarean (Arn; Bell-p; Calen; Caust; Cham; Hyp; Phos; Sec; Staph)
- Retention of urine[3,6,9,12,13] (Acon; Arn; Ars; Bell; Caust; Hyp; Lyc; Sec; Staph)
- Shock (emotional)[8] (Acet-ac; Acon; Arn; Hyp; Ign; Phos; Rescue remedy; Staph)
- Spontaneous abortion[2,8,9,12,13] (Acon; Alet; Apis; Arn; Bell; Caul; Cimic; Ferr; Goss; Helon; Ip; Kali-c; Kali-p; Nux-v; Puls; Sab; Sec; Sep)
- Subinvolution[8] (Arn; Bell; Bry; Calc; Carb-v; Caul; Chin; Cimic; Goss; Helon; Puls; Sab; Sec; Sep; Staph; Ust)
- Vaginal bleeding during pregnancy (Acon; Arn; Bell; Caul; Ign; Kali-c; Kali-p; Puls; Sab; Sec; Sep; Tril)

Phosphorus (Phos). Other names: White phosphorus

Prime indications:
- **Very anxious and fearful**
- **Oversensitive to all external impressions**
- **Very imaginative**
- **Marked thirst for ice cold drinks which may be vomited as soon as they become warm in the stomach**
- **Empty feeling in the epigastrium or entire abdomen**
- **Ravenous hunger with faintness or fainting from hunger or hungry at night and after meals**
- **Burning pains and sensations of heat**
- **Worse lying on the left side**

Additional characteristics:
General
- Lacking in vitality
- Easily catches colds leading to respiratory troubles
- Sensitive to noise or strong odours, which may cause fainting
- Haemorrhages, with tendency to bleed from every mucous surface and every body orifice
- Bruises easily[4]
- Vertigo

Emotional
- Nervous and restless
- Perceptive
- Fear of death or being alone
- Mental dullness with weak memory

Caused by
- Loss of vital fluids
- Strong emotions
- Mental exertion
- Getting wet
- Tobacco

Sensations
- Emptiness, especially in the head[4]

- Heaviness
- Numbness
- Fullness
- Coldness in certain parts
- The palms of the hands are hot

Pains
- Burning
- Pressing
- Stitching

Worse
- Evening
- Cold
- Night
- Thunderstorms
- Motion

Better
- Warmth
- Eating

Notes
- Phosphorus must not be used before or after Causticum
- Phosphorus follows well after Bryonia, Calcarea carbonica, China, Kali carbonicum or Lycopodium
- Phosphorus is followed well by Belladonna, Nux vomica or Silica

Suggested uses:
- After pains felt in the sacrum
- Anaemia[1,6,10,11] (Alet; Ars; Calc; Carb-v; Cinn; Cupr; Ferr; Helon; Ign; Kali-c; Kali-p; Merc; Nat-m; Puls; Sab; Sep; Staph; Sul-ac; Tril)
- Backache[3,6,8] (Bell; Bry; Calc; Cimic; Ferr; Hyp; Kali-c; Kali-p; Lyc; Merc; Nat-m; Nux-v; Puls; Sep; Sil; Zinc)
- Constipation during pregnancy[6,10,11,12] (Caust; Collins; Cupr; Graph; Kali-c; Lyc; Mag-m; Mag-p; Nux-v; Op; Puls; Sep)
- Diarrhoea[3,8,9,10,12] (Ars; Chin; Merc; Puls) during pregnancy
- Excessive lactation[2,6,9] (Bell; Bor; Bry; Calc; Cham; Con; Lac-c; Lyc; Phyt; Ust)
- Fear[1,4,6] (Arg-n; Ars; Calc; Cimic; Gels; Ign; Op; Puls; Rescue remedy)
- Gestational hypertension[3] (Acet-ac; Apis; Ars; Bell; Calc; Ferr; Gels; Helon; Kali-c; Lyc; Merc; Nat-m; Op; Puls; Sep; Zinc)
- Ill effects of general anaesthetic[7] (Acet-ac; Nux-v; Op)
- Inadequate lactation[2,6] (Acon; Arg-n; Apis; Ars; Bell; Bry; Calc; Caust; Cham; Dulc; Graph; Ign; Lyc; Phyt; Puls; Sil; Urt-u)
- Mastitis[1,9] (Acon; Ars; Apis; Arn; Bell; Bry; Calc; Cham; Con; Graph; Lac-c; Lyc; Merc; Phyt; Puls; Sil)
- Nausea and vomiting[2,5,6,7,8,9] (Acet-ac; Alet; Ant-t;

Chel; Goss; Ip; Nux-v; Puls; Sep). Unable to drink water during pregnancy, as this causes vomiting. May feel nauseous when placing her hands in warm water and must close her eyes while bathing, as even the sight of water may cause vomiting
- Neonatal jaundice[3,6,11] (Acon; Ars; Bry; Cham; Chel; Chin; Mag-m; Merc; Nux-v; Sep)
- Postpartum haemorrhage[4,6,7,8,10,11,12] (Acet-ac; Acon; Bell; Bry; Carb-v; Caul; Chin; Cinn; Ferr; Ham; Ip; Kali-c; Sab; Sec; Sep; Ust)
- Proteinuria[2,3,8,9,11,12] (Apis; Ars; Bell; Ferr; Gels; Helon; Kali-c; Lyc; Merc; Nat-m; Sab; Sep)
- Recovering after caesarean[3,7] (Arn; Bell-p; Cham; Hyp; Op; Sec; Staph)
- Shock (emotional) (Acet-ac; Acon; Arn; Hyp; Ign; Op; Staph; Rescue remedy)
- Sleeplessness in infants[8] (Acon; Bell; Cham; Puls)
- Sore, cracked nipples[1] (Acet-ac; Acon; Arn; Ars; Bell; Calc; Cast-eq; Caust; Cham; Graph; Hyp; Lac-c; Lyc; Merc; Phyt; Puls; Sep; Sil; Staph; Rescue remedy)

Phytolacca (Phyt) *Phytolacca decandra.* Other names: Poke root, Virginian poke, target weed, pigeon berry, American nightshade

---

Prime indications:
- **Pains changing location rapidly**
- **Worse in cold, damp weather**
- **Glands affected**

Additional characteristics:
General
- Rheumatic, feeling exhausted, stiff and worn-out
- Oversensitive to pain, which feels intolerable
- Unable to drink hot fluids
- Vertigo, with dimness of vision

Emotional
- Melancholy
- Indifferent
- Irritable
- Fearful, that she is sure to die
- May become shameless

Sensations
- Of lump in the throat

Pains
- Like electric shocks
- Shifting position
- Soreness all over

Worse
- Rising from bed
- Motion
- Night

Better
- Cold drinks
- Lying on abdomen
- Warmth

Note Phytolacca follows well after Bryonia

Suggested uses:
- Breast-feeding problems with pain radiating all over the body[4]
  - Mammary abscesses
  - Mastitis[6,9,10,11] (Acon; Ars; Apis; Arn; Bell; Bry; Calc; Cham; Con; Graph; Lac-c; Merc; Puls; Sil)
  - Sore, cracked nipples (Bell; Calc; Cast-eq; Caust; Cham; Graph; Lyc; Phos)
- Excessive lactation[2] (Bell; Bor; Bry; Calc; Cham; Con; Lac-c; Phos; Ust)
- Inadequate lactation[2] (Acon; Apis; Arg-n; Ars; Bell; Bry; Calc; Caust; Cham; Dulc; Graph; Ign; Lyc; Phos; Puls; Sil; Urt-u)
- Ligament pain[3]/sciatica[6,8,10,12] (Arn; Bell-p; Caust; Ferr; Mag-p; Puls; Sep) where pains run from the hip downward, mostly on the outward side of the thighs
- Regulation of milk supply in general[4] (Bell; Calc; Puls; Sil)
- Sore, cracked nipples[3,4,6,12] (Acet-ac; Acon; Arn; Ars; Bell; Calc; Cast-eq; Caust; Cham; Graph; Hyp; Lac-c; Lyc; Merc; Phos; Puls; Sep; Sil; Staph; Rescue remedy)

Pulsatilla (Puls) *Pulsatilla nigricans.* Other names: Meadow anemone, European windflower, pasque flower, anemone pratensis

---

Prime indications:[7]
- **Mild, yielding disposition**
- **Tendency to weep and apologize for taking so long**
- **Worse in a warm room and in the evening**
- **Relieved by cold applications and open air**
- **Thirstless, even though mouth is dry**
- **Changeable**

Additional characteristics:
General
- Finds the room hot and stuffy and wants the window open
- Faintness and fainting
- Chilliness
- Vertigo
- Discharges from mucous membranes thick and yellow
- Symptoms erratic and changeable
- Symptoms occur on one side of the body only

Emotional
- Changeable and easily moved to laughter or tears
- Affectionate
- Suspicious

- Wants sympathy and responds well to it
- Wants company and invites lots of people to the birth
- Wants to be touched
- Anxious restlessness with fear of being alone, going insane or the dark
- Dullness
- Indifference
- Hysteria

Sensations
- Numbness of single parts or affected part
- Pulsations
- Heat

Pains
- Cutting
- Stitching
- Tearing
- Pressing
- Wandering

Worse
- Evening
- Before midnight
- Getting feet wet
- Warmth
- Standing or lying down

Better
- Cold
- Cold applications
- Open air
- Pressure
- Gentle motion

Notes
- Pulsatilla follows Apis, Bryonia, Calcarea carbonica, Chamomilla, Lycopodium, Nux vomica or Silica well
- Pulsatilla is followed well by Chamomilla or Graphites

Suggested uses:
- Abdominal pain[7,8] (Acet-ac; Arn; Ars; Cupr; Nux-v; Sep; Staph) from motions of fetus
- After pains[2,3,8,9] (Arn; Caul; Cham; Cimic; Cupr; Hyp; Mag-p; Nux-v; Sab; Sec; Sil)
- Anaemia[5,6,7,13] (Alet; Ars; Calc; Carb-v; Chin; Cupr; Ferr; Helon; Kali-c; Kali-p; Merc; Nat-m; Phos; Staph; Sul-ac; Tril)
- Backache[3,8] (Bell; Bry; Calc; Cimic; Ferr; Hyp; Kali-c; Kali-p; Lyc; Merc; Nat-m; Nux-v; Phos; Sep; Sil; Zinc)
- Constipation during pregnancy[5,7,8,12] (Caust; Collins; Cupr; Graph; Ign; Kali-c; Lyc; Mag-m; Mag-p; Nux-v; Op; Phos; Sab; Sep)
- Depression[2,4,7] (Chin; Cimic; Con; Ign; Nat-m; Sep)
- Diarrhoea[2,3,4,5,6,7,8,9,12] (Ars; Chin; Merc; Phos) from fright during pregnancy

- Dizziness and fainting during pregnancy[7,8,9,10,12] (Ars; Bell; Cimic; Gels; Ign; Kali-c; Laur; Nat-m; Nux-v; Sep)
- Eye discharges in infants[7,8,9,11] (Acon; Apis; Arg-n; Ars; Bell; Bry; Calc; Lyc; Nat-m; Zinc)
- Failure to progress[1,3,6,7,9,12,13] (Acon; Arn; Bell; Bor; Carb-v; Caul; Cham; Chin; Cimic; Cinn-m; Coff; Cupr; Gels; Ign; Kali-c; Kali-p; Lyc; Mag-m; Nat-m; Nux-v; Op; Sec; Sep)
- Fear[1,4,7] (Acon; Arg-n; Ars; Calc; Cimic; Gels; Ign; Op; Phos; Rescue remedy)
- Frequency of micturition[3,8,9,12] (Ars; Bell; Caust; Nat-m; Sep)
- Gestational hypertension[3] (Acet-ac; Apis; Ars; Bell; Calc; Ferr; Gels; Helon; Kali-c; Lyc; Merc; Nat-m; Op; Phos; Sep; Zinc)
- Haemorrhoids[1,2,3,6,7,8,9,11] (Ars; Collins; Ham; Hyp; Ign; Kali-c; Lyc; Nat-m; Nux-v; Sab; Sep; Staph), especially postpartum
- Heartburn[2,5,6] (Acet-ac; Bry; Calc; Carb-v; Caust; Merc; Nat-m; Zinc)
- Hypertension during labour[2] (Acon; Apis; Arn; Bell; Cham; Cimic; Gels; Ign; Merc; Nat-m; Op; Sep)
- Inadequate lactation[2,3,6,8,9] (Acon; Apis; Arg-n; Ars; Bell; Bry; Calc; Caust; Cham; Dulc; Graph; Ign; Lyc; Phos; Phyt; Sil; Urt-u)
- Insomnia[2,3,7,8,12] (Acon; Bell; Bell-p; Coff; Con; Gels; Ign; Kali-c; Nux-v; Op)
- Ligament pain/sciatica[8,10] (Arn; Bell-p; Caust; Ferr; Mag-p; Phyt; Sep)
- Malposition[4,6,8,9]/malpresentation.[9,13] Used for turning breech or transverse presentation if no other remedy is indicated and the woman feels well. However, to work efficiently, the remedy must be given before the presenting part becomes engaged or fixed in the pelvis (e.g. week 35 or 36) or before the membranes are ruptured[13]
- Mastitis[7,9] (Acon; Apis; Ars; Arn; Bell; Bry; Cham; Con; Graph; Lac-c; Lyc; Merc; Phos; Phyt; Sil)
- Nausea and vomiting[2,3,5,6,7,8,9,12] (Acet-ac; Alet; Ant-t; Ars; Chel; Goss; Ip; Nux-v; Phos; Sep)
- Pain relief during labour (Acon; Arn; Bell; Caul; Cham; Cimic; Coff; Cupr; Gels; Ign; Kali-c; Lyc; Mag-m; Mag-p; Nux-v; Sec; Sep)
- Postnatal depression[6,8] (Chin; Cimic; Con; Ign; Nat-m; Sep)
- Proteinuria[3,12] (Apis; Ars; Bell; Gels; Helon; Kali-c; Lyc; Merc; Nat-m; Phos; Sab; Sep)
- Regulate milk supply[4,6] (Bell; Calc; Phyt; Sil). To dry up milk after weaning[2,3]
- Retained placenta[2,3,6,8,9,13] (Bell; Caul; Cimic; Goss; Ign; Nux-v; Sab; Sec; Sep) following labour if there are no indications for another remedy
- Sleeplessness in infants[8] (Acon; Bell; Cham; Phos)

- Sore, cracked nipples[2,4] (Acet-ac; Acon; Arn; Ars; Bell; Calc; Cast-eq; Caust; Cham; Graph; Hyp; Lac-c; Lyc; Merc; Phos; Phyt; Sep; Sil; Staph; Rescue remedy)
- Spontaneous abortion[7,8,9,12,13] (Acon; Alet; Apis; Arn; Bell; Caul; Cimic; Ferr; Goss; Helon; Ip; Kali-c; Kali-p; Nux-v; Op; Sab; Sec; Sep; Tril) in weeks 32–36[9]
- Subinvolution[8] (Arn; Bell; Bry; Calc; Carb-v; Caul; Chin; Cimic; Goss; Helon; Op; Sab; Sec; Sep; Staph; Ust)
- Vaginal bleeding during pregnancy (Acon; Arn; Bell; Caul; Ign; Kali-c; Kali-p; Op; Sab; Sec; Sep; Tril)
- Vaginal discharge and candida during pregnancy[2,7] (Bor; Helon; Merc; Nat-m; Sep)
- Varicose veins[5,6,7,8,9] (Bell-p; Calc; Carb-v; Ferr; Ham; Lyc; Nux-v; Puls; Sep; Tril; Zinc) in upper and lower limbs

Bach Flower Rescue Remedy

Discovered by Dr Edward Bach in the 1930s, the Bach Flower Remedies are not, strictly speaking, homeopathic remedies in that their mode of preparation and means of selection and application are different. They are designed to act primarily on negative emotions and promote peace of mind. Rescue remedy is a combination of several Bach Flower remedies and has been briefly described here as many women choose to include it in their labour kit to help them cope with any anxieties they (or their birthing partner) may experience during labour.

Rescue remedy is a combination of the following:

- Star of Bethlehem for shock
- Rock Rose for terror, fear and panic
- Impatiens for mental and physical tension where the person is unable to relax and is agitated and irritable
- Cherry Plum for loss of emotional control, where the person becomes hysterical with much screaming and shouting
- Clematis for the bemused feeling which often precedes a faint.

Prime indications:
- **Emotional shock**
- **Fear and anxiety**
- **Panic**
- **Insomnia due to anxiety and fear**
- **Fainting from fright**
- **Before, during or after labour**

For the above, a few drops of the remedy are dropped directly onto the tongue when needed or added to a glass of water and sipped frequently. If it is preferred that the mother does not drink, a few drops can be added to her bath or rubbed gently behind her ears and on her wrists and temples.

Other uses:
- Painful/tender nipples
- Cracked nipples
- Bruising and physical trauma following delivery
- Rashes

In these situations, Rescue remedy can be applied to the affected area neat or in cream form as often as required. Rescue remedy cream contains Crab Apple as an additional ingredient to those listed above and acts on feelings of self-hatred or a sense of uncleanliness. In the case of tender or cracked nipples, the cream may be applied directly before or after feeding as it is quick-drying and non-greasy and will not have any adverse effect on the baby.

Secale (Sec) *Secale cornutum*, containing the fungus *Claviceps pupurea*, ergot. Other names: Ergot of rye

Prime indications:
- **Great objective coldness, but worse from covering**
- **Restlessness**
- **Passive haemorrhage**

Additional characteristics:
General
- Emaciated and feeble multiparae
- Cold
- Rapidly sinking in strength
- Skin may be dry, harsh and wrinkled
- Evidence of peripheral vasospasm especially in trunk and limbs

Emotional
- Shameless

Caused by
- Lifting
- Suppression of lochia, milk or sweat

Sensations
- Numbness and tingling
- Internal heat, external coldness

Pains
- Burning

Worse
- Warmth
- Warm room
- Least motion
- Being covered

Better
- Uncovering
- Cold applications

Suggested uses:
- After pains[2,6,7,8,11,12,13] (Arn; Caul; Cham; Cimic; Cupr; Hyp; Kali-c; Mag-p; Nux-v; Puls; Sab; Sil) too severe and long-lasting
- Colic (Cham; Cupr; Ign; Ip; Mag-m; Mag-p; Nux-v; Staph)
- Ill effects of syntometrine
- Failure to progress[3,6,7,9,12,13] (Acon; Arn; Bell; Bor; Carb-v; Caul; Cham; Chin; Cimic; Cinn-m; Coff; Gels; Kali-c; Kali-p; Lyc; Mag-m; Nat-m; Nux-v; Op; Puls; Sep). Pains weak, irregular or have ceased with no expulsive action taking place, even though everything appears open and loose
- Pain relief during labour[3] (Acon; Arn; Bell; Caul; Cham; Cimic; Coff; Cupr; Gels; Ign; Kali-c; Lyc; Mag-m; Mag-p; Nux-v; Puls; Sep)
- Postpartum haemorrhage[2,4,6,7,8,10,11,12,13] (Acet-ac; Acon; Bell; Bry; Carb-v; Caul; Chin; Cinn-m; Ferr; Ham; Ip; Kali-c; Phos; Sab; Sep; Ust) copious, dark, watery and offensive. Accompanied by tingling in the hands and constant spreading apart of the fingers
- Prolonged lochia (Calc; Caul), offensive,[12,13] fetid[6] and thin or accompanied by prolonged bearing down pains[12]
- Puerperal mania[13] (Ars; Bell; Cimic; Cupr; Lyc; Zinc)
- Recovering from caesarean (Arn; Bell-p; Cham; Hyp; Op; Phos; Staph)
- Retained placenta[1,2,6,7,8,9] (Bell; Caul; Cimic; Goss; Ign; Nux-v; Puls; Sab; Sep) from uterine inertia or hour-glass constriction
- Retention of urine[7,12] (Acon; Arn; Ars; Bell; Caust; Hyp; Lyc; Op; Staph)
- Spontaneous abortion[1,2,3,5,6,7,8,9,11,12,13] (Acon; Alet; Apis; Arn; Bell; Caul; Cimic; Ferr; Goss; Helon; Ip; Kali-c; Kali-p; Nux-v; Sab; Sep; Tril) in 12th week
- Subinvolution[2,8] (Arn; Bell; Bry; Calc; Carb-v; Caul; Chin; Cimic; Goss; Helon; Op; Puls; Sab; Sep; Staph; Ust)
- Suppression or drying up of milk[9,11] (Bell; Puls)
- Vaginal bleeding during pregnancy (Acon; Arn; Bell; Caul; Ign; Kali-c; Kali-p; Op; Puls; Sab; Sep; Zinc)

Sepia (Sep) *Sepia officinalis*. Other names: Cuttlefish ink

Prime indications:[7]
- **Sad, weeping, irritable, quarrelsome and averse to company, yet may dread to be alone**
- **Indifference and loss of affection for their nearest and dearest**
- **Yellow saddle across upper part of cheeks and nose**
- **Bearing down sensation in abdomen, relieved by sitting with limbs crossed**
- **Empty 'gone' sensation in epigastrium**

- **Chilly, made worse by becoming heated**
- **Better from vigorous exercise**
- **Stagnation and burnout**

Additional characteristics:
General
- Exhausted and run down by the pressures of responsibility
- Perspires easily and profusely
- Extremely sensitive to the cold
- Weakness
- Faintness and fainting
- Trembling
- Restless
- Does not tolerate pressure of clothing
- Craves sour foods, e.g. lemons, vinegar
- Marked aversion to fat

Emotional
- Does not tolerate contradiction
- Impatient
- Frightened easily
- Confused and mentally dull
- Hysterical
- Does not tolerate noise

Caused by
- Anger
- Grande multiparity
- Loss of vital fluids
- Suppressed sweat

Sensations
- Coldness or numbness of single parts
- Dragging down
- Emptiness
- Heaviness
- As of a ball in inner parts

Pains
- Stitching
- Shooting upwards

Worse
- Cold air
- Thunderstorms
- Consolation

Better
- Vigorous exercise
- Sun
- Cold bathing

Notes
- Sepia follows well after Natrum muriaticum, Nux vomica or Silica
- Sepia is followed well by Nux vomica

Suggested uses:
- Abdominal pain[6,8,13] (Acet-ac; Arn; Ars; Cupr; Nux-v; Puls; Staph) due to fetal movements
- Anaemia[3] (Alet; Ars; Calc; Carb-v; Chin; Ferr; Helon; Kali-c; Kali-p; Merc; Nat-m; Phos; Puls; Staph; Sul-ac; Tril)
- Backache[3,7,8,12] (Bell; Bry; Calc; Cimic; Ferr; Hyp; Kali-c; Kali-p; Lyc; Merc; Nat-m; Nux-v; Phos; Puls; Sil; Zinc)
- Carpal tunnel syndrome[8] (Apis; Ars; Calc; Caust; Lyc)
- Constipation during pregnancy[2,3,5,7,8,9,10,11,12] (Caust; Collins; Cupr; Graph; Ign; Kali-c; Lyc; Mag-m; Mag-p; Nux-v; Op; Phos; Puls; Sab)
- Cramping[1,3,8,9] (Calc; Cham; Cupr; Ferr; Ign; Mag-p; Nux-v; Zinc)
- Delayed recovery (Carb-v)
- Depression[7] (Chin; Cimic; Con; Ign; Nat-m; Puls)
- Dizziness and fainting during pregnancy[7,8,9,12] (Ars; Bell; Cimic; Gels; Ign; Kali-c; Laur; Nat-m; Nux-v; Puls)
- Failure to progress[9,13] (Acon; Arn; Bell; Bor; Carb-v; Caul; Cham; Chin; Cimic; Cinn-m; Coff; Cupr; Gels; Ign; Kali-c; Kali-p; Lyc; Mag-m; Nat-m; Nux-v; Op; Puls; Sec)
- Frequency of micturition[6,8,11,12] (Ars; Bell; Caust; Nat-m; Puls)
- Gestational hypertension[3] (Acet-ac; Apis; Ars; Bell; Calc; Ferr; Gels; Helon; Kali-c; Lyc; Merc; Nat-m; Op; Phos; Puls; Zinc)
- Haemorrhoids[2,3,7,8,11] (Ars; Collins; Ham; Hyp; Ign; Kali-c; Lyc; Nat-m; Nux-v; Puls; Sab; Staph)
- Hair loss after giving birth[2] (Calc; Carb-v; Lyc; Nat-m; Sil)
- Hypertension during labour (Acon; Apis; Arn; Bell; Cham; Cimic; Gels; Ign; Merc; Nat-m; Op; Puls)
- Ligament pain/sciatica[6,7,8] (Arn; Bell-p; Caust; Ferr; Mag-p; Phyt; Puls)
- Loss of libido[2,7,8,12] (Caust; Graph; Nat-m)
- Nausea and vomiting[2,3,4,6,7,8,9,12,13] (Acet-ac; Alet; Ant-t; Ars; Chel; Goss; Ip; Nux-v; Phos; Puls) made worse by the smell of food, but relieved by eating
- Neonatal jaundice[3,6,8] (Acon; Ars; Bry; Cham; Chel; Chin; Mag-m; Merc; Nux-v; Phos)
- Pain relief[3] (Acon; Arn; Bell; Caul; Cham; Cimic; Coff; Cupr; Gels; Ign; Kali-c; Lyc; Mag-m; Mag-p; Nux-v; Puls; Sec)
- Postnatal depression[6] (Chin; Cimic; Con; Ign; Nat-m; Puls)
- Postpartum haemorrhage[7,8,13] (Acet-ac; Acon; Bell; Bry; Carb-v; Caul; Chin; Cinn-m; Ferr; Ham; Ip; Kali-c; Phos; Sab; Sec; Ust)
- Proteinuria[8,9] (Apis; Ars; Bell; Ferr; Gels; Helon; Kali-c; Lyc; Merc; Nat-m; Phos; Sab)
- Pruritus vulvae[2,3,6,9,10,11] (Acon; Ars; Bell; Bor; Calc; Coff; Collins; Graph; Ham; Helon; Lyc; Merc; Sil)
- Retained placenta[6,8,13] (Bell; Caul; Cimic; Goss; Nux-v; Puls; Sab; Sec), especially following spontaneous abortion if there are no indications for another remedy
- Sore, cracked nipples[1,3,6,9,12,13] (Acet-ac; Acon; Arn; Ars; Bell; Calc; Cast-eq; Caust; Cham; Graph; Hyp; Lac-c; Lyc; Merc; Phos; Phyt; Puls; Sil; Staph; Rescue remedy)
- Spontaneous abortion[2,3,5,6,7,8,9,12,13] (Acon; Alet; Apis; Arn; Bell; Caul; Cimic; Ferr; Goss; Helon; Ip; Kali-c; Kali-p; Nux-v; Op; Puls; Sab; Sec Tril) between 20–36 weeks
- Subinvolution[2,3,7,8] (Arn; Bell; Bry; Calc; Carb-v; Caul; Chin; Cimic; Goss; Helon; Op; Puls; Sab; Sec; Staph; Ust)
- Vaginal bleeding during pregnancy (Acon; Arn; Bell; Caul; Ign; Kali-c; Kali-p; Op; Puls; Sec; Tril)
- Vaginal candida during pregnancy (Bor; Helon; Merc; Nat-m; Puls)
- Varicose veins[6,7] (Bell-p; Calc; Carb-v; Ferr; Ham; Lyc; Nux-v; Puls; Tril; Zinc) on the legs and around the ankles. The legs feel heavy, as if paralysed, stiff and unwieldy, especially in the morning after sleep. Varices may also appear on the genitals during pregnancy

---

Silica (Sil). Other names: Flintstone, mountain crystal, silicea, silicon dioxide, SiO_2

Prime indications:[7]
- **Defective assimilation of nutrition**
- **Exhaustion**
- **Induration**
- **Suppuration**
- **Perspiration of single parts**
- **Chilly, worse from cold and better from heat**
- **Discharges are foul, offending and offensive**

Additional characteristics:
General
- Lacks 'grit', weak, nervous and sensitive
- Dry skin
- Catches colds easily
- Oversensitive to pain
- Constipated, with difficulty expelling stool
- Restless

Emotional
- Mild
- Lacking in confidence
- Morose
- Obstinate
- Difficulty in concentrating

Caused by
- Lifting
- Suppression of foot sweat

Sensations
- Numbness of single parts
- Heaviness (internal or external)
- As of a hair

Pains
- Sharp
- Tearing
- Sore
- Pressing

Worse
- Evening and night
- Cold
- Motion
- Touch or being jolted
- Pressure
- Lying on painful side
- Mental effort
- Consolation

Better
- Warmth
- Wrapping up

Notes
- Silica follows well after Belladonna, Bryonia, Calcarea carbonica, Graphites, Ignatia, Lycopodium or Phosphorus
- Silica is followed well by Lycopodium, Pulsatilla or Sepia
- Mercurius should not be given before or after Silica

Suggested uses:
- After pains[8] (Arn; Caul; Cham; Cimic; Cupr; Hyp; Mag-p; Nux-v; Puls; Sab; Sec)
- Backache[3,6,8] (Bell; Bry; Calc; Cimic; Ferr; Hyp; Kali-c; Kali-p; Lyc; Merc; Nat-m; Nux-v; Phos; Puls; Sep; Zinc)
- Constipation[3,4,6,7,8,10,11,12] (Calc; Caust; Graph; Kali-c; Lyc; Nux-v; Op; Phos; Puls; Sep) in infants and during pregnancy
- Hair loss after giving birth[2,3,6] (Calc; Carb-v; Lyc; Nat-m; Sep)
- Infected umbilical cord[4] (Calen)
- Inverted nipples or ulceration of nipples, with sharp pain in breast.[6] Inflamed nipples having a darting or burning pain
- Sore, cracked nipples[3,8,12] (Acet-ac; Acon; Arn; Ars; Bell; Calc; Cast-eq, Caust; Cham; Graph; Hyp; Lac-c; Lyc; Merc; Phos; Phyt; Puls; Sep; Staph; Rescue remedy)
- Mastitis[4,9,11] (Cham; Graph; Phyt; Puls), deep red in the centre and rose-coloured towards the periphery. Swollen, hard and very sensitive. The constant burning pain prevents rest
- Milk refused by the infant. The quality of the milk is such that the infant vomits after nursing
- Pruritus vulvae[6,9] (Acon; Ars; Bell; Bor; Calc; Coff; Collins; Graph; Ham; Helon; Lyc; Merc; Sep)
- Regulation of milk supply[4,6,9] (Bell; Bry; Calc; Cham; Lyc; Phos; Phyt; Puls)

Staphysagria (Staph) *Delphinium staphysagria*. Other names: Stavesacre, Palmated larkspur

Prime indications:
- **Suppressed emotions, especially anger and indignation**
- **Hypersensitive physically and emotionally**
- **Worse after afternoon nap**
- **Suffers pain acutely, out of proportion to the injury**

Additional characteristics:
General
- Dislikes milk, tobacco, water

Emotional
- May appear pleasant and compliant on the outside, but resentment is building up within them, together with a sense of violation or humiliation, which is finally released in a violent outburst
- Violently angry, throwing things
- Anxious about others
- Apathetic
- Capricious
- Disappointed
- Forgetful
- Irritable
- Resentful
- Offended easily

Pains
- Tearing, especially in nerve-rich parts of body

Caused by
- Unexpressed anger or indignation
- Difficult or assisted delivery
- Episiotomy
- Surgery
- Accident

Sensation
- Of a ball in the forehead

Worse
- Exertion
- Fasting
- Touch
- Pressure

Better
- Warmth
- Rest

Suggested uses:
- Abdominal pains during pregnancy which come on suddenly, e.g. after an unexpected kick from the baby (Acet-ac; Arn; Ars; Cupr; Nux-v; Puls; Sep). There may be shock and/or anger

- Anaemia (Alet; Ars; Calc; Carb-v; Chin; Ferr; Helon; Kali-c; Kali-p; Merc; Nat-m; Phos; Puls; Sep; Sul-ac; Tril) with gums pale and bleeding
- Caesarean, after[2,3,12] (Arn; Bell-p; Cham; Op; Phos; Sec)
- Catheterization, after[4]
- Colic[5,12] (Cham; Cupr; Ign; Ip; Mag-m; Mag-p; Nux-v; Sec) with cramping after drinking, due to anger or indignation
- Haemorrhoids following difficult labour[3] (Ars; Collins; Ham; Hyp; Ign; Kali-c; Lyc; Nat-m; Nux-v; Puls; Sab; Sep)
- Retention of urine[4,12] (Acon; Arn; Ars; Bell; Caust; Hyp; Op; Sec) after forceps delivery

- Shock (emotional)[8] (Acet-ac; Acon; Arn; Hyp; Ign; Op; Phos; Rescue remedy)
- Sore, cracked nipples[4] (Acet-ac; Acon; Arn; Ars; Bell; Calc; Cast-eq; Caust; Cham; Graph; Hyp; Lac-c; Lyc; Merc; Phos; Phyt; Puls; Sep; Sil; Rescue remedy). Retracted[3]
- Subinvolution[8] (Arn; Bell; Bry; Calc; Carb-v; Caul; Chin; Cimic; Goss; Helon; Op; Puls; Sab; Sec; Sep; Ust)
- Wounds or injuries with feelings of humiliation, indignation or anger. This may occur when there has been more surgical intervention than expected, after painful assisted delivery or unpleasant or painful internal examination

REFERENCES

1. Allen T F 1990 The encyclopedia of pure materia medica – a record of the positive effects of drugs upon the healthy human organism. Jain, New Delhi
2. Boericke W 1988 Pocket manual of homoeopathic materia medica comprising the characteristic and guiding symptoms of all remedies, 9th edn. Jain, New Delhi
3. Boger C M 1996 A synoptic key of the materia medica. Jain, New Delhi
4. Borland D M 1950 Homoeopathy for mother and infant. British Homoeopathic Association, London
5. Clarke J H 1987 The prescriber, 9th edn. C W Daniel, Saffron Walden
6. Clarke J H 1991 Dictionary of homoeopathic materia medica (3 vol), 3rd edn. Homoeopathic Book Service, Sittingbourne
7. Farrington H 1991 Homoeopathy and homoeopathic prescribing. Jain, New Delhi
8. Kunzli von Fimmelsberg J 1987 Kent's repertorium generale. Jain, New Delhi
9. Knerr C B 1992 Repertory of Hering's guiding symptoms of our materia medica. Jain, New Delhi
10. Nash E B 1986 Leaders in homeopathic therapeutics, 4th edn. Insight Editions, Worthing
11. Neatby E A, Stonham T G 1990 A manual of homoeotherapeutics – an introduction to the study and practice of homoeopathy, 3rd edn. Foxlee-Vaughan, London
12. Von Lippe A 1991 Key notes and red line symptoms of the materia medica. Jain, New Delhi
13. Yingling W A 1989 Accoucheur's emergency manual. Jain, New Delhi

FURTHER READING

Bach E 1931 Heal thyself. C W Daniel, Saffron Walden
Bach E 1933 The twelve healers and other remedies. C W Daniel, Saffron Walden
Burnett V R, Brown L K eds 1993 Myles textbook for midwives, 12th edn. Churchill Livingstone, Edinburgh
Castro M 1992 Homoeopathy for mother and baby: pregnancy, birth and the postnatal year. Macmillan, London
Howard J 1990 The Bach flower remedies step by step. C W Daniel, Saffron Walden
Jansen J W 1992 Synthetic bedside repertory for gestation, childbirth and childhood. Merlijn, Haarlem
Moskowitz R 1992 Homoeopathic medicines for pregnancy and childbirth. North Atlantic Books, Berkley
Murphy R 1993 Homoeopathic medical repertory – a modern repertory. Hahnemann Academy of North America, Pagosa Springs, Colorado

Phatak S R 1977 Materia medica of homeopathic medicines. Indian Books and Periodicals Syndicate, New Delhi
Phatak S R 1977 A concise repertory of homoeopathic medicines, 2nd edn. Homeopathic Medical Publishers, Bombay
Schroyens F 1993 Synthesis – repertorium homoeopathicum syntheticum. Homoeopathic Book Publishers, London
Sweet B, Tiran D 1996 Mayes' Midwifery, 12th edn. Baillière Tindall, London
Tiran D, Mack S 1995 Complementary therapies for pregnancy and childbirth. Baillière Tindall, London
Tyler M L 1987 Homeopathic drug pictures. C W Daniel, Saffron Walden
Vermeulen F 1992 Synoptic materia medica. Merlijn, Haarlem

Part 7

Appendices

Appendix 1
remedy pictures (other remedies)

Acetic acidum (Acet-ac). Other names: Acetic acid, $HC_2H_3O_2$

- Anaemia with oedema
- Chilly
- Craves fat and salt
- Weak
- Difficulty breathing
- Profuse perspiration
- Irritable
- Worried about business affairs

Worse: Night; after eating
Better: Lying on the stomach; day; during rest

Uses:
- Anaemia[6]
- Cracked nipples[4]
- Emotional shock following surgery[12]
- Gestational hypertension, oedema[3]
- Heartburn[2,8] during pregnancy
- Ill effects of anaesthesia[12]
- Nausea with sour belching and vomiting[2]
- Postpartum haemorrhage[13] with great thirst, not relieved by drinking

Aletris farinosa (Alet) *Aletris farinosa*. Other name: Stargrass

- Anaemic, tired all the time
- Great weakness
- Confusion
- Inability to concentrate
- Fainting with vertigo.

Uses:
- Anaemia[6,13]
- Nausea and vomiting during pregnancy[6,8]
- Spontaneous abortion[6,8]

Argentum nitricum (Arg n). Other names: Silver nitrate, Ag NO$_3$

- Anxious unrest
- Nervous excitement
- Anxiety causes rapid motion
- Anticipatory apprehension and fear with diarrhoea

Worse: Mental exertion; sweets/sugar; night; 11 am; crowded room; warmth; emotional excitement; after eating
Better: Cold air; open air; eructations; heavy pressure

Uses:
- Anticipatory anxiety[6]
- Discharges from the eye in infants[5,8,9] of thick yellow mucus or pus
- Fear during pregnancy and labour, with hurry[4] and must walk and walk
- Urinary incontinence[11]

Borax veneta (Bor). Other names: Sodium biborate, tincal

- Breast-feeding mothers and breast-fed infants
- Tearful at night, scream during their sleep
- Fear of downward motion, therefore dislike being rocked or put down in their cot
- Irritable, especially before passing stool or micturating
- Easily startled by noise

Worse: Cold; travelling in a car; lying on right side
Better: Fresh air; pressure on painful part

Uses in mother:
- Pain in opposite breasts during or after breast-feeding[6]
- Breasts aching when empty[6]
- Candida and vaginal discharge during pregnancy[2,3,6,8]
- Excessive lactation[2]
- Failure to progress[13] with contractions darting upward
- Pruritus vulvae[2,6,9]

Uses in baby:
- Candida of the mouth and/or tongue[1,5,8,10] so tender that the child is prevented from feeding

Castor equi (Cast-eq) *Equus caballus*. Other name: Rudimentary thumb-nail of the horse

Where there are no symptoms indicative of another remedy, used for:

- Sore, cracked nipples, very tender, cannot bear the touch of clothing.[1] With burning and itching[2,9]

- Breasts swollen and tender, worse descending the stairs.[6] A sensation as if the breasts would fall off causes the woman to press her hands against them. Worse left breast[9]

Collinsonia canadensis (Collins) *Collinsonia canadensis*. Other name: Stone root

- Pelvic and portal congestion
- Emotionally gloomy

Worse: Slightest mental emotion or excitement; cold; night; pregnancy
Better: heat

Uses:
- Constipation[6] during third trimester[2,5,8,9,11]
- Haemorrhoids[2,3,6,8,9,10,11] with inertia of the lower bowel[9]
- Pruritus vulvae[2,6,9,11] especially late in pregnancy. Sore, can only sit on the very edge of a chair[9]

Conium (Con) *Conium maculatum*. Other names: Poison hemlock, poison parsley

- Depressed from overexcitement or strain
- Weak memory
- Timid and afraid of being left alone
- Vacant expression, with no interest in anything

Worse: Lying down
Better: Sitting

Uses:
- After pains extending from left to right when baby put to the breast
- Breast-feeding problems with breasts hard, lumpy and painful. Stitching pains in nipples. The woman wants to press the painful breast hard with her hand
- Depression (postnatal)
- Excessive lactation.[2,9] May be used to dry up milk after weaning[2]
- Insomnia
- Mastitis[6,11]

Cuprum (Cupr) *Cuprum metallicum*. Other names: Copper, Cu

- Spasms and cramps
- Coldness and blueness of face and body

Worse: During pregnancy; hot weather; touch
Better: Cold drinks; perspiring

Uses:
- After pains especially in multiparae,[6,13] extending to calves and soles of feet[2]
- Anaemia[11]
- Colic
- Constipation[8,11]
- Cramping in the calves and legs during pregnancy.[1,2,3,6,8,11] Worse during coitus
- Failure to progress during labour
- Pain relief during labour
- Puerperal mania, with violent delirium[5,6]

Dulcamara (Dulc) *Solanum dulcamara*. Other names: Bittersweet, woody nightshade

- Catches cold easily
- Restless and impatient
- Wants many different things which are rejected as soon as they are obtained

Worse: Cold and damp
Better: Motion; warmth

Uses:
- Absence of milk[6,8] due to a cold
- Backache (lumbar), with difficulty walking[6]
- Cystitis
- Spontaneous abortion following exposure to the cold and damp

---

Ferrum (Ferr) *Ferrum metallicum*. Other names: Iron, Fe

- Anaemic due to faulty assimilation of iron
- Vasomotor imbalance
- Haemorrhage
- Anxious from slightest cause
- Excited easily
- Angered by least contradiction
- Wants to be alone

Worse: Sitting; perspiring; after cold washing; after over-heating; midnight and towards morning
Better: Gentle motion; after rising

Uses:
- Anaemia[5,11]
- Backache during pregnancy[8]
- Cramping in calves, soles and toes[5,8,11]
- Ligament pain/sciatica[8]
- Postpartum haemorrhage,[2,3,10,11,13] bright red, coagulates easily. With dark clots[3]
- Proteinuria[3,9]
- Spontaneous abortion[1,8,10,13]
- Varicose veins in the legs[8,9]

Gossypium (Goss) *Gossypium herbaceum*. Other name: Cotton plant

- Promotes firm, regular and strong uterine contractions
- Similar to Cimicifuga in action

Worse: Motion; pressure; before breakfast
Better: Rest

Uses:
- Acceleration of labour
- Failure to progress during labour with feeble, near painless contractions and exhaustion[9]
- Morning sickness followed by faintness[3,6]
- Retained placenta especially after premature labour[2,13]
- Spontaneous abortion[6,13]
- Subinvolution

Hamamelis (Ham) *Hamamelis virginica*. Other names: Witch hazel, spotted alder, winter bloom, snapping hazelnut

- Venous problems with prickling and stinging pains
- Great sensitivity to touch
- Engorgement
- Inflammation
- Relaxation of veins in any part of the body

Worse: Pressure; cold air; being jolted; motion; touch; night
Better: Resting

Uses:
- Bruised soreness of abdominal wall during pregnancy[6]
- Haemorrhoids[2,5,6,10,11] especially during puerperium[9]
- Passive uterine haemorrhage[2,6,10,11]
- Phlegmasia alba dolens[6]
- Pruritus vulvae[11]
- Sore nipples[6]
- Varicose veins[2,5,6,8,9,12] of the legs where there are no clear indications for another remedy. The veins become hard, knotty, swollen and painful with cramping pain at night preventing sleep[13]

Helonias (Helon) *Helonias dioica*. Other name: Unicorn root

- Anaemic[6,13] and easily fatigued
- Probable history of several spontaneous abortions
- Irritable, melancholy and wants to be left alone

Worse: Motion; contradiction
Better: Occupation

Uses:
- Candida[2,8] vaginal discharge during pregnancy

- Proteinuria during pregnancy[6,8,9]
- Pruritus vulvae[2,6,9] with irritation of external labia, which are puffed, red, itching and burning
- Sore, cracked nipples.[6,9] Cannot bear the touch of clothing
- Spontaneous abortion[8,10,13]
- Subinvolution[2]

Hypericum (Hyp) *Hypericum perforatum*. Other names: St John's wort, 'Arnica of the nerves'

An ingredient in Hypercal tincture, a few drops of which are added to a glass of water and then applied directly to wounds to aid healing and reduce pain.

- Wounds extremely sensitive to touch
- Puncture wounds
- Wounds of parts rich in nerves – brain, spine, coccyx and finger ends
- After instrumental delivery
- Nervous depression following wounds, surgery, shock or fright

Worse: Motion; touch; pressure; night
Better: Lying quietly

Uses:

- After pains – violent in sacrum and hips[6,8,9,13] with severe headache[9]
- Back pain following forceps delivery,[6] epidural, injury to coccyx, with severe headache[8,9,13]
- Catheterization, after
- Haemorrhoids[11]
- Retention of urine after labour[13] with soreness of the urethra
- Shock[6,8]
- Sore, cracked nipples[13]

Ignatia (Ign) *Ignatia amara*. Other name: St Ignatius bean

- Alternating mental states, e.g. sadness, weeping to involuntary laughter
- Suited to sensitive, excitable, nervous
- Gentle, refined and overconscientious

Worse: Emotional excitement; mental exertion; consolation; touch
Better: Change of position; while eating; hard pressure; warmth

Uses:

- Colic, especially in breast-fed infant whose mother is grieving[9]
- Constipation[8,11]
- Cramping

- Depression (postnatal)[5,6] following worry, grief, fright or disappointment
- Fear during pregnancy and labour[1,4,6,9,11]
- Failure to progress[13]
- Haemorrhoids,[6,11] following labour,[8] better walking. Pain when sitting and standing and/or stitching pain during cough
- Hypertension during labour[2]
- Inadequate lactation[8,9]
- Insomnia.[5,9] Restless, dream-filled sleep, hearing everything
- Pain relief during labour
- Pruritus vulvae where itching extends up into the vagina
- Retained placenta[2]
- Shock (nervous)[3,8]
- Spontaneous abortion[13] accompanied by weeping

Lac caninum (Lac-c) *Canis familiaris*. Other name: Bitches' milk

---

- Alternation of symptoms from side to side[13]
- Relief of pain by cold applications or uncovering
- Vertigo with floating sensation
- Very low self-esteem
- Forgetful and absent-minded
- Fears being alone

Worse: Touch; being jolted; pressure; during rest; at night
Better: Open air; turning on the right side; walking

Uses:

- Excessive lactation without any known cause[2,9]
- Mastitis[6] so sore and painful that the woman holds her breasts to stop them moving, with constant pain in the nipples
- To dry up milk after weaning[2,9]
- Weeping while breast-feeding

Laurocerasus (Laur) *Prunus laurocerasus*. Other name: Cherry laurel

---

- Lack of reaction, especially in chest and heart complaints
- Slow, weak, irregular pulse
- Cold, clammy, pale or cyanosed
- Eyes staring and wide open

Worse: Sitting up; before eating; least exertion; evening
Better: Night; open air; lying down

Uses:

- Asphyxia neonatorum with cyanosis.[4,8,10,13] The baby's face is blue, the muscles of the face twitch and the baby gasps for air. Its breathing is almost

imperceptible or panting. No mechanical obstruction (meconium aspiration). With white body and blue head and extremities[14]
- Dizziness and fainting[6]

Magnesia muriatica (Mag-m). Other names: Chloride of magnesium, $MgCl_2$

- Rushed and hurried, needs to be doing something all the time
- Made worse from mental exertion
- History of indigestion or uterine disease

Worse: Night; after drinking milk; noise; lying on the right side
Better: Fresh air; hard pressure; gentle motion

Uses:
- Colic in babies, caused by teething or milk. Indigestion, green diarrhoea or constipation with small, crumbling, sheep dung-like stools[5,9]
- Constipation during pregnancy[6,10,11]
- Failure to progress[13]
- Infant is unable to digest milk, which passes undigested
- Insomnia due to restless anxiety in bed on closing the eyes. May be unable to go to sleep due to oversensitivity to noise
- Pain relief during labour

Magnesia phosphorica (Mag-p). Other names: 'Homeopathic aspirin', phosphate of magnesium, $MgHPO_47H_2O$

- Remedy almost specific to pain
- Sharp, piercing or violent cramp-like pains
- Spasmodic contraction of muscles
- Sensitive and nervous
- Complaints occur on the right side of the body

Worse: Motion; light touch; cold; being uncovered; walking in fresh air
Better: Heat; pressure; friction; hot bath

Uses:
- Catheterization, after
- Colic with eructations of gas, causing infant to bend double[6,10]
- Constipation during pregnancy
- Cramping in the calves[2,5,6]
- Ligament pain/sciatica[6,8]
- Pain in ovaries and uterus forcing the woman to bend double
- Pain relief during labour

- Sciatica where pains shoot from the sciatic notch to the popliteal space or the heel

Mercurius (Merc) *Mercurius vivus*, Hg. Other names: Quicksilver or ammonio-nitrate of mercury (which are indistinguishable in their action) Mercurius solubilis $[2(NH_2Hg_2)NO_3H_2O]$

- Perspiration easy, offensive and does not relieve
- Children with unusually large heads, slow in reaching developmental milestones

Worse: Night; wet weather; warmth of bed; open air; motion; during sleep
Better: Getting out of bed in the morning

Uses:
- Anaemia[11]
- Backache during pregnancy[8]
- Breast abscesses
- Candida[1,8] with profuse salivation and slimy diarrhoea[3,5,6,10,11]
- Diarrhoea[3,4,6] during pregnancy
- Eye discharges in infants[6,8,9] of yellow mucus or pus
- Gestational hypertension,[3] especially oedema
- Heartburn where stomach feels empty, with hiccups and burping[8]
- Hypertension during labour
- Mastitis.[9] The infant rejects the milk[6]
- Neonatal jaundice[5,6,9,11]
- Proteinuria[2,3,8,11]
- Pruritus vulvae[2,6,9,11]
- Sore, cracked nipples[4,6] on attempting to breast-feed
- Vaginal discharge/candida[2,6]

Sabina (Sab) *Juniperus sabina*. Other name: Savine

- Profuse haemorrhage, bright red, gushing and mixed with dark red or black clots. Fluid blood and clots in equal parts[9]
- Made worse by least motion.[6,13] Accompanied by drawing labour-like pains from the sacrum or small of the back to the pubes. Pains in the joints may accompany the flow[13]

Worse: Warmth
Better: Open air; walking about[13]

Uses:
- After pains,[2,3,6,8,11,13] intense with discharge of bright red blood with clots and pain as described above
- Constipation[3,11]
- Haemorrhoids[2,11] bleeding[3]
- Postpartum haemorrhage as described above[2,3,6,11]
- Proteinuria[2]

- Premature labour[2]
- Retained placenta,[2,6,8,13] especially following spontaneous abortion[9] with intense pain and abdomen sensitive to touch
- Secondary postpartum haemorrhage, 8 days after labour[9]
- Spontaneous abortion at 12–16 weeks,[2,3,5,6,8,10,11,13] with copious brown haemorrhage[14] and diarrhoea
- Subinvolution[8] with continued bleeding where there are no clear indications for another remedy

Sulphuricum acidum (Sul-ac), H_2SO_4. Other names: Sulphuric acid, oil of vitriol

- Anaemic and exhausted
- Chilly
- Internally hurried, causing everything to be done 'at a pace' in spite of exhaustion

Worse: Heat; evening; mid-morning
Better: Warmth

Uses:
- Anaemia[13]
- Bruises which do not heal in spite of trying Arnica[8]
- Oral candida in infants, on tongue and gums[1,6,8,10]

Trillium pendulum (Tril) *Trillium pendulum.* Other name: White beth root

- bright red haemorrhage accompanied by faintness, anxious restlessness and vertigo

Worse: Overexertion; after eating
Better: Bending forward; open air

Uses:
- Anaemia[13]
- Incontinence[8]
- Postpartum haemorrhage[2,6] with a sensation that the pelvis will fall apart, which is made better by tight bandaging
- Spontaneous abortion[6,8,9,13] between 8–16 weeks
- Varicose veins during pregnancy, especially in the legs and ankles[8,13]

Urtica urens (Urt-u) *Urtica urens.* Other name: Common nettle

Uses:
Where there are no symptoms indicative of another remedy, Urtica urens is useful for regulating the milk supply.

- Establishing a good supply of milk in the early days of feeding, where it is slow without obvious cause[6,9]
- Breast-feeding problems where the milk supply is either low[5,8] or overabundant for the baby's demand[6]
- To dry up milk after weaning[2,6,8,9]

Worse: Being cool
Better: Rubbing; lying down

Ustilago (Ust) *Ustilago maidis.* Other names: Corn smut

Uses:
- Passive haemorrhage after delivery or spontaneous abortion[13] occurring between 12–16 weeks. Intermittent[13]
- Blood oozes, forming long, black clots[13]
- Excessive lactation[2,6,9] accompanied by depression. With shooting pains down the thighs or under left breast
- Secondary postpartum haemorrhage, 2 weeks after labour[9]
- Subinvolution.[2,6,8] Uterus feels drawn into a knot

Zincum (Zinc) *Zincum metallicum.* Other names: Zinc, Zn.

- Run down by stress or overwork
- Face may be alternately pale then red
- May be depressed or irritable
- Twitching and restless legs in spite of exhaustion

Worse: Night; touch; wine
Better: Motion; while eating

Uses:
- Backache during pregnancy[8,10]
- Constipation in the newborn in nervous, twitchy babies who scream on waking[6]
- Cramping in the calves during pregnancy[1]
- Eye discharges in infants[6]
- Gestational hypertension
- Heartburn with sweetish eructations[8,9]
- Inadequate lactation[6,9]
- Puerperal mania[2]
- Spontaneous abortion[5,6,9]
- Taste in the mouth, metallic or bloody[8,9]
- Varicose veins of leg, thigh and/or vulva[2,6,8,12]

REFERENCES

1. Allen T F 1990 The encyclopedia of pure materia medica – a record of the positive effects of drugs upon the healthy human organism. Jain, New Delhi
2. Boericke W 1988 Pocket manual of homeopathic materia medica comprising the characteristic and guiding symptoms of all remedies, 9th edn. Jain, New Delhi
3. Boger C M 1996 A synoptic key of the materia medica. Jain, New Delhi
4. Borland D M 1950 Homoeopathy for mother and infant. British Homoeopathic Association, London
5. Clarke J H 1987 The prescriber, 9th edn. C W Daniel, Saffron Walden
6. Clarke J H 1991 Dictionary of homoeopathic materia medica (3 vol), 3rd edn. Homeopathic Book Service, Sittingbourne
7. Farrington H 1991 Homeopathy and homeopathic prescribing. Jain, New Delhi
8. Kunzli von Fimmelsberg J 1987 Kent's repertorium generale. Jain, New Delhi
9. Knerr C B 1992 Repertory of Hering's guiding symptoms of our materia medica. Jain, New Delhi
10. Nash E B 1986 Leaders in homoeopathic therapeutics, 4th edn. Insight Editions, Worthing
11. Neatby E A, Stonham T G 1990 A manual of homoeotherapeutics – an introduction to the study and practice of homoeopathy, 3rd edn. Foxlee-Vaughan, London
12. Von Lippe A 1991 Key notes and red line symptoms of the materia medica. Jain, New Delhi
13. Yingling W A 1989 Accoucheur's emergency manual. Jain, New Delhi

Appendix 2
remedy abbreviations for suggested uses in Part 6

Abbreviation	Full name	Official name
Acet-ac	Acetic acidum	Acetic acid
Acon	Aconite	*Aconitum napellus*
Alet	Aletris farinosa	*Aletris farinosa*
Ant-t	Ant tart	*Antimonium tartaricum*
Apis	Apis	*Apis mellifica*
Arg-n	Argentum nitricum	Silver nitrate
Arn	Arnica	*Arnica montana*
Ars	Arsenicum	Arsenicum album
Bell	Belladonna	*Atropa belladonna*
Bell-p	Bellis	*Bellis perennis*
Bor	Borax veneta	Sodium biborate or tincal
Bry	Bryonia	*Bryonia alba*
Calc	Calcarea carb	Calcarea carbonica
Calen	Calendula	*Calendula officinalis*
Carb-v	Carbo veg	Carbo vegetabilis
Cast-eq	Castor equi	Equus caballus
Caul	Caulophyllum	*Caulophyllum thalicroides*
Caust	Causticum	Causticum hahnemanni
Cham	Chamomilla	*Matricaria chamomilla*
Chel	Chelidonium	*Chelidonium majus*
Chin	China	*China officinalis* or *Cinchona calisaya*
Cimic	Cimicifuga	*Cimicifuga racemosa* or *Actaea racemosa*
Cinn-m	Cinnamomum	*Cinnamomum majus*
Collins	Collinsonia	*Collinsonia canadensis*
Coff	Coffea	*Coffea cruda* or *Coffea arabica*
Con	Conium	*Conium maculatum*
Cupr	Cuprum	Cuprum metallicum
Dulc	Dulcamara	*Solanum dulcamara*
Ferr	Ferrum	Ferrum metallicum
Gels	Gelsemium	*Gelsemium sempervirens*
Goss	Gossypium	*Gossypium herbaceum*
Graph	Graphites	Plumbago

Remedy abbreviations for suggested uses in Part 6 (*cont'd*)

Abbreviation	Full name	Official name
Ham	Hamamelis	*Hamamelis virginica*
Helon	Helonias	*Helonias dioica*
Hyp	Hypericum	*Hypericum perforatum*
Ign	Ignatia	*Ignatia amara*
Ip	Ipecac	*Cephaelis ipecacuanha*
Kali-c	Kali carb	Potassium carbonicum or Potassium carbonate
Kali-p	Kali phos	Potassium phosphoricum or Potassium phosphate
Lac-c	Lac caninum	*Canis familiaris*
Laur	Laurocerasus	*Prunus laurocerasus*
Lyc	Lycopodium	*Lycopodium clavatum*
Mag-m	Magnesia muriatica	Chloride of magnesium
Mag-p	Magnesia phosphorica	Phosphate of magnesium
Merc	Mercurius	Mercurius vivus or Mercurius solubilis
Nat-m	Nat mur	Natrum muriaticum or Sodium chloride
Nux-v	Nux vomica	*Strychnos nux vomica*
Op	Opium	*Papaver somniferum*
Phos	Phosphorus	Phosphorus
Phyt	Phytolacca	*Phytolacca decandra*
Puls	Pulsatilla	*Pulsatilla nigricans*
Sab	Sabina	*Juniperus sabina*
Sec	Secale	*Secale cornutum*
Sep	Sepia	*Sepia officinalis*
Sil	Silicea	Silicon dioxide
Staph	Staphysagria	*Delphinium staphysagria*
Sul-ac	Sulphuricum acidum	Sulphuric acid
Tril	Trillium pendulum	*Trillium pendulum*
Urt-u	Urtica urens	*Urtica urens*
Ust	Ustilago	*Ustilago maidis*
Zinc	Zincum	Zincum metallicum

Appendix 3
Glossary of homeopathic terms

Aggravation The temporary worsening of symptoms which may occur a short time after taking a remedy.

Centesimal The scale of dilution 1:100, denoted as C.

Complementary remedy One that is 'harmonious' in action when given before or after a chosen remedy.

Constitution The overall state of health including temperament, character, personal history, past medical history and treatment, inherited tendencies, lifestyle and reaction to environmental factors.

Constitutional remedy Remedy selected during constitutional treatment, which takes into account all of the above factors.

Constitutional treatment Rather than acting on the presenting symptoms alone, the aim is to treat the whole person by taking into account all the factors given above (see *Constitution*), along with the local symptoms of the disease.

Dynamis Another term for 'vital force'.

Isopathy Technique of prescribing in which the remedy is made from the causative agent of a disease.

Laws of Cure Originally described by Constantine Hering, these principles govern the healing process as it is frequently seen during constitutional treatment. As someone is cured their symptoms move from the innermost organs to the outermost (i.e. from the most important to life to the less important); from the top of the body downwards (e.g. from the head to the hands and feet); in reverse order of their appearance in the history of the case.

Materia Medica Detailed descriptions of homeopathic remedies with their associated symptoms and uses.

Miasm The term Hahnemann used to describe the basic underlying cause of chronic and recurrent disease conditions – a block to health which is usually inherited or may be acquired after contracting a disease. Of most relevance during constitutional treatment.

Modalities The factors that qualify a particular symptom, e.g. pain better from applied heat.

Mother tincture The starting material for a homeopathic remedy, normally with a mixture of water and alcohol as solvent, before the process of potentization. Available from homeopathic pharmacies. Most useful in first aid situations where a few drops of tincture are added to water before applying to the cut, burn, etc.

Nosodes Remedies made from disease products, diseased tissue or pathogenic organisms.

Picture The summary of the symptoms, mental states and pathological changes that a substance is able to cause in the healthy and therefore can cure in the sick.

Polycrest A remedy which has a rich symptom picture and a wide range of clinical application. Such a remedy is well known and will most often be used for constitutional treatment.

Polypharmacy Technique of prescribing in which two or more remedies are given simultaneously, either as a combined formula or in alternation with one another.

Potency The strength of a remedy according to the number of times it has been diluted and succussed. A potency having undergone six successive stages of dilution and *succussion* on the centesimal scale is written 6C. Generally low potency = 1X to 12X or 6C; medium potency = 30C; high potency = 200C to 1M, 10M and beyond.

Potentization The process of making a homeopathic remedy by repeated dilution and *succussion*.

Proving The means of testing potential homeopathic remedies. Healthy volunteers (provers) take repeated doses of a substance until symptoms are produced. These are then noted for eventual inclusion in the *Materia Medica* and *Repertory*.

Repertory Index of symptoms, with each symptom heading or rubric listing remedies known to cause the symptom. Used in conjunction with the *Materia Medica*.

Sarcodes Remedies made from potentized glands and their secretions, e.g. Thyroidinum, Adrenalin, etc.

Similimum That remedy which matches the symptom picture of the patient most closely.

Specific remedy One which is given for a particular problem without taking into account the whole person, as the sphere of action of the remedy is limited, e.g. *Castor equi* for sore, cracked nipples.

Succussion The vigorous shaking that accompanies each stage of dilution during the preparation of a homeopathic remedy.

Susceptibility Vulnerability to disease.

Symptom picture The range of symptoms experienced by a person, including mental, emotional, general and physical symptoms. Required to make the closest match with a remedy.

Tautopathy A variant on *isopathy* which refers specifically to the prescription of a potentized drug or toxin that a person has ingested at some time in the past.

Trituration The process of grinding an insoluble substance with saccharin lactose during the preparation of a potency.

Universal remedy Another term for *polycrest*.

Vital force The term Hahnemann used to describe the energy governing the recuperative powers of the human body. A return to health can only be brought about by returning the vital force to a state of well-being.

Appendix 4
Useful addresses

FURTHER INFORMATION

For more information about homeopathy and homeopathic training contact:

Society of Homoeopaths
2 Artizan Road, Northampton NN1 4HU
Tel: 01604 21400

Institute of Complementary Medicine
PO Box 194, London SE16 1QZ
Tel: 0171 237 5165

Hahnemann Society
Humane Education Centre, Bounds Green Road, London N22 4EU

Faculty of Homoeopathy
The Royal Homoeopathic Hospital, Great Ormond Street,
London WC1N 3HR
Tel: 0171 837 8833

London College of Classical Homoeopathy
Hahnemann House, 32 Welbeck Street, London WIM 7PG
Tel: 0171 487 4322

Research Council for Complementary Medicine (RCCM)
5th Floor, 60 Great Ormond Street, London WC1 3JF
Tel: 0171 833 8897

British Complementary Medicine Association
St Charles Hospital, Exmoor Street, London W10 6DZ
Tel: 0181 964 1205

British Homoeopathic Association
27a Devonshire Street, London W1
Tel: 0171 935 2163

HOMEOPATHIC LIBRARY INFORMATION SERVICE

Hom-inform
Faculty of Homoeopathy, Glasgow Homoeopathic Hospital, 1000 Great Western Road, Glasgow G12 0NR
Tel: 0141 211 1617
Fax: 0141 211 1610

BOOKSHOPS

Ainsworths and Helios Homoeopathic Pharmacies and the British Homoeopathic Association have book lists of homeopathic books and operate a mail order service (see list of homeopathic pharmacies). The Homoeopathic Supply Co, which also operates a mail order service, stocks selected titles on self-development, general and specialist homeopathy and provings.

Homoeopathic Supply Co.
Fairview, 4 Nelson Road, Sheringham, Norfolk NR26 8BU
Tel: 01263 824683
Fax: 01263 821507

A comprehensive selection of books on homeopathy, including those published abroad, can be obtained from:

Minerva Books
173 Fulham Palace Road, London W6 8QT
Tel: 0171 385 1361

HOMEOPATHIC PHARMACIES

Most are happy to give advice and will also have a 24-hr telephone answering service for orders. Remedies will be sent out with an invoice.

Ainsworths Homoeopathic Pharmacy
36, New Cavendish Street, London W1M 7LH
Tel: 0171 935 5330 (24-hr answering service)

Galen Homoeopathics
Lewell, Dorchester, Dorset
Tel: 01305 263996 (24-hr answering service)

Gould's Homoeopathic Chemist
14 Crowndale Road, London NW1
Tel: 0171 388 4752 (daytime number) or 0171 387 1888

Helios Homoeopathic Pharmacy
97 Camden Road, Tunbridge Wells, Kent TN1 1QR
Tel: 01892 536393 (24-hr answering service) or 01892 537254 (9.30 am–5.30 pm)

Weleda Homoeopathic Pharmacy
Weleda (UK) Ltd, Heanor Road, Ilkeston, Derbyshire DE7 8DR
Tel: 01602 309 319 (24-hr answering service)

FURTHER INFORMATION ON BACH FLOWER REMEDIES CAN BE OBTAINED FROM:

Dr Edward Bach Centre
Mount Vernon, Sotwell,
Wallingford, Oxon OX10 0PZ
Tel: 01491 834 678

Bach Flower Remedies Customer Enquiries
Broadheath House, 83 Parkside, Wimbledon, London SW19 5LP

Index

Printed in the United Kingdom
by Lightning Source UK Ltd.
125989UK00001B/56/A